Firm Roots—Strong Limbs

Firm Roots—Strong Limbs

G. Ray Pharr

iUniverse, Inc.
New York Lincoln Shanghai

Firm Roots—Strong Limbs

iUniverse books may be ordered through booksellers or by contacting:

iUniverse
2021 Pine Lake Road, Suite 100
Lincoln, NE 68512
www.iuniverse.com
1-800-Authors (1-800-288-4677)

ISBN: 0-595-34358-9

Printed in the United States of America

Contents

PROLOGUE

If *there is no rest for the wicked and the righteous don't need it*, then where does Ray J. fit in? Here he thought he had the whole summer to relax and catch up on his loafing, and now his son, John, arrives with his wife with an assignment for him to do.

They barely get out of the drive to return to California when Ray J. complains to his wife, Joan.

"Those two daughters of his must have been born with questions on the brain. I have never known anyone to ask so many of them. I think we all did a pretty good job of raising them after their mother took off that way. Apparently the older one is satisfied, but the younger one has never felt completely safe. I guess most of us would be a little insecure if we had never known our mothers and had to rely on heresy about them.

"It seems her latest series of questions have been about his background, and even mine, for she wants to know all about where we came from and what we did before she was born. He has tried to answer her questions, but he doesn't know that much about anything that happened before he was born.

"He thinks I have nothing to do in the summers but play golf all day, so I should take the time to write all this stuff down and send it to him."

◆ ◆ ◆

"Well, son, I hardly know where to begin. (But, first, let me tell you. I'm not that good with words so if I borrow a few phrases from somebody else, I will put them into italics).

"As I reflect upon my childhood, I was the ham within the sandwich of my family: three siblings older, three siblings younger, with only one of them a girl. As a teenager my mother told me of having had three boys, and when I arrived as the fourth, she began to think she would never have

1

a daughter. In short order after me she has two miscarriages and then finally a daughter; seven years later, two more boys with only two years between them.

"With so many children, Mother has to have help in keeping the house clean and one maid is just not sufficient. Lawrence, the oldest, sweeps the floors, and Nick makes the beds. Doug, the scoundrel, always works harder at keeping out of work than the work itself would have required. It falls my lot to help with the cooking and washing of clothes.

"Little did I know back then what these early chores would do for me in my adult life. My first wife would be a registered nurse who had to wear heavily starched uniforms, so I had to sprinkle them down and iron them. My second wife still gets embarrassed when I tell how I was in the garage one day during our first year of marriage and opened a box from the shelf to discover a box of my wrinkled shirts crammed into it. Confronting her with it, she admits how she hates to iron. She has been buying new ones and hiding these from me. Never have understood why anyone hates ironing; gives a body something to do while his mind wanders.

"Now if my wife, my kids, my grandkids, and even my great grandkids read this, I can hear them saying:

'So his mind started to wander way back then'?"

1920's

North Carolina

Origin of the Tree

Even in North Carolina in the late 1800's, everyone had heard the jokes about the farmer's daughter, but Noah Robbins knows that Margaret is far from being the farmer's daughter that the jokes apply to. She is somewhat pale, but her eyes make him forget the color of her skin or the frailness of her body; she is that awesome in his sight. Noah is twenty-one and Margaret is only seventeen when they run away and get married. He brings her to the old homestead that his father left him when he died.

When he asks her to marry him, he tells her,

"There's no mortgage on this land; this land is ours—all four hundred fifty acres. We will grow tobacco, cotton, corn, and wheat. We will have cattle in the pasture my daddy fenced, and we will raise pigs so we will have ham for breakfast. We'll raise chickens to have eggs to go with the ham and meat to eat for supper. I've already planted a garden with lettuce, tomatoes, corn, peas, beans, turnips, and squash."

◆　　　◆　　　◆

Long ago, his grandfather had dug two wells, one near the house and another in the bottomland. He wanted one near his work so he wouldn't waste time in climbing the hill to get a drink of water. Had he only known the price that climb would cost in later years!

Margaret gives birth to Leola before they celebrate their first anniversary and in so doing almost loses her life. Noah vows she will never have another child; no child can possibly mean as much to him as Margaret does. He hires a local widow to come in to look after Margaret and Leola while he works the farm.

Tall, with broad shoulders and strong legs, Noah walks behind a plow driven by a mule from sunup to sundown. He has a deep, bass voice and sings as he plows—loud enough that Margaret can hear him whenever he bursts into song. While growing up he sang hymns, but after marrying Margaret, he sings only love songs, pouring out his heart for her.

For five blissful years, Noah gets up at dawn and slips out to milk the cow and feed the pigs and chickens before coming back into the house for breakfast. Margaret brushes her hair, long wavy hair that has never been cut, and dresses before coming downstairs to fry ham and eggs with home-made biscuits for their breakfast.

Leola sleeps until her daddy has already left the house to work all day in the fields, and her mother has gone back to bed to finish her sleep. Most of her days are spent in the company of the widow who looks after her.

Martha, the widow, is fairly tall for a woman and she is young; no lines under her eyes even though she cried for months after lightning killed her husband. Her skin is smooth and soft. Her hair is simply done, parted in the middle and tied in a loose knot on the nape of her neck. She has small delicate features and a kindly look about her. She takes Leola's education upon herself and at an early age teaches her to read and write.

It is July, the day is hot and humid, and Noah spends the day in the bottomland working among tall corn. Trying to finish one more patch of corn, he stays late and gets so thirsty that he takes the lid off the old well and brings up water in a bucket tied to a rope. By the time he gets to the house, he has a fever that never goes down. He dies of typhoid fever.

Knowing it would worry him, Margaret is four months pregnant and doesn't let Noah know about it. When Noah dies, she gives up the will to live and goes to bed until Earl is born. When she refuses to get up, her brother Willie comes over at once.

"Margaret, you must get up; you have two children to look after."

"Brother, you have to look after them because I want to be with my husband. My love for him is far greater than my love for the children, and I don't want to live without him."

With that said, she closes her eyes and dies. The doctor is called, and when he examines her, he finds nothing wrong so he puts on her death certificate that she died of a broken heart.

◆   ◆   ◆

Kindly Aunt Bessie Blankenship, Leola's great aunt on her mother's side, takes the two children into her small home. Aunt Bessie is a little, shriveled woman with a face filled with wrinkles and pale blue eyes. Her hair is long, wrapped around her head and held in place with Bobbie pins. She has a shy manner and a gentle voice. She knows nothing about children, but she is anxious to do her duty. Her husband, Uncle Quince, is so indifferent, so selfish, but she knows in her heart of his indifference and loves him humbly all the same.

"Dear, I know this is a tiny room for you to share with little Earl, but it's the best I have. Look, there is a large tree just outside your windows."

The windows are small, narrow, and very little light comes through. Dark draperies are over them, dusty from hanging so long. An air of deep irredeemable gloom hangs over the room. Leola still bears a memory of the many solemn hours she spends in this room during the year with Aunt Bessie.

It is late, almost bedtime for young Earl, when Uncle Willie brings his bride, Aunt Molly, to visit them. He has spent the past year finishing his education at a seminary over in Virginia. He takes Leola by the hand and leads her around the house to sit on the front porch. For a moment, he stands before her. He is a tall man, bony, with straw-colored hair, a pale face and blue eyes that shine as he gazes at her. He puts his hands in his pockets and says to her:

"I wonder what kind of life you will lead. What will happen to shape you into the person that one day you will become? You haven't had much love and attention up to now, but I will do my best to make amends from now on. I have finished my study in the seminary and have a home to bring you and Earl into. Your Aunt Molly and I cannot be the parents you once had, but we will do the best we can. Your daddy's place is just across the hill from mine; one day it will be yours and Earl's."

Heavy rains the night before have swollen the streams they are to cross to get home. Uncle Willie stops the horse on the wooden bridge and speaks quietly as the horse dances nervously about. The moon has come out from behind the clouds and the wind blows across the water, making small waves. The timbers of the bridge begin to crack dangerously and the horse jumps forward, but Uncle Willie gains control of the frightened horse, and they get home before the rain starts again.

Leola climbs the stairs slowly, finds her room and listens. She has never had a room all her own. She is a little frightened as she closes the door behind her. The bed is made, and a nightgown is lying on the pillow. She climbs up on the bed and puts her head on the pillow and lies quite still.

◆   ◆   ◆

Aunt Molly is different. Her hair is elaborately dressed, with a curl in the middle of her forehead. It is black, shiny black, and twisted into a knot at the back of her head. Her eyes are almost black, and there is a slight crook in her long nose. She smiles a great deal, but her mouth is wide, and she tries to hide her large teeth which are somewhat yellow.

Most of Leola's early years are spent looking after her brother Earl, and then in six short years she has Demie, Eva, Lena, and Belle to care for. Uncle Willie teaches at the local high school during the week and preaches on Sunday at Rose Chapel Baptist Church.

Having four daughters in such a short time has taken its toll on Aunt Molly. She has migraine headaches and spends a lot of time in a dark room or in bed with the covers over her head, leaving all five kids in Leola's care.

Earl is a frail child and is little trouble during his teenage years. He has few friends for his habit of reading isolates him; he soon grows tired and listless when in the company of others. When he first goes to school, he is humiliated when the other boys laugh at his use of big words, which he never overcomes, so he remains shy and silent until he graduates.

His love for Leola remains steadfast throughout his life. His quiet manner helps both of them when she has a tooth that abscesses and Uncle Willie isn't home. Earl heats his pocketknife to kill the germs on it, rubs whiskey on her gums, and cuts out the infection.

The oldest daughter, Demie, has a pretty face and abundant dark hair. From the moment she begins to walk, she follows Leola everywhere she goes. She crawls upon her lap and begs her to read to her. Leola teaches her to read before she starts to school. No surprise that these two will become schoolteachers when they grow up.

Eva, the second daughter, is tall and thin and somewhat of a tomboy. She spends most of her time climbing trees and taking long walks down in the pasture along the riverbanks. Leola spends more time trying to keep track of where she is than she spends reading to Demie.

Shorter than the others and with a tendency to be chubby, Lena sneaks into the cookie jar every chance she gets so Leola hides it in different places. Uncle Willie has a "sweet tooth" so Leola likes to keep fresh cookies for him whenever he comes home.

From birth, Belle is the beauty of the family: creamy skin, naturally curly black hair, a smile always on her face; everyone wants to play with her. She begins to walk at an early age and is always skipping and playing near the house, singing every song she hears on the radio.

◆   ◆   ◆

Convinced that God is calling him to spread His Word, Uncle Willie quits his teaching position, withdraws all the money he has saved, and buys a large tent. His gifts are great. He has a fine presence and great learning with a voice that is powerful, melodious, and eloquent.

The Sunday that he opens his tent in a little community of Olin, more than two hundred people come to hear him preach. Word soon spreads to other communities and "Uncle Willie" becomes a household name throughout the county.

As Uncle Willie becomes more involved in his preaching and having revival meetings that last a week at a time, he spends less time at home. Aunt Molly gets worse in her resentment of having so many children in the house with all the noise that makes her headaches worse. She becomes more vocal in expressing her anger, especially toward Leola and Earl.

"Without you two", she tells Leola, "we would have more money to spend on buying nice clothes for my own daughters. I'm tired of doing without so many things we could have if we didn't have you. Your own mother didn't love you enough to fight for her life, so why should we do without for you?"

Of course when Uncle Willie is home on weekends, she is still the sweet aunt that she wants him to observe. Leola vows:

"Whenever I get married and have children, my husband and I will love them enough to do without any material things."

But she never "talks back" to Aunt Molly. Uncle Willie impresses respect for elders upon them. When he is before his congregation, he preaches hell and damnation; but, at home with the kids, he is kind and gentle, teaching them quietly how to be ladies and a gentleman.

> *The Spirit of God Is Within Each of Us*
> *Love Thy Neighbor As Thyself*
> *Don't Let The Sun Go Down On Your Wrath*
> *Judge Not!*
> *But The Greatest Gift From God Is Love, So Always Say:*
> *I Love You*

Finishing at the local school, Demie wants to become a teacher, but the closest college is almost fifty miles away. Uncle Willie prays and prays about her leaving home at such a young age, but he wants her to be educated. When Leola tells them that she, too, wants to become a teacher,

Aunt Molly reminds her that they have little money to pay for her expenses.

"And you haven't got any money," she says.

"I'm going to sell the jewelry my parents left."

She inherited from her parents a gold watch and chain, two rings, two pins, and a pearl broach. When Aunt Bessie hears that she is going to sell those things, she goes to the bank immediately and withdraws her savings.

Handing the envelope to Leola, she shyly says:

"It's a little present I have for you. I couldn't bear the thought that you would sell the few things you have that were once your parents."

"Dear Aunt Bessie. I can't possibly take this from you. It is so good of you to offer, but I can't accept it."

"Please take it. It will make me happy if you do."

"But you will need it sooner or later."

"No. I don't think I will ever need it. I was keeping it in case Quince died before me, but I don't think I will live very much longer now."

"Please don't say that, Aunt Bessie. You will live for a number of years more."

"I'm not sorry." Her voice almost breaks, but she smiles and continues:

"I used to pray that God would not take me first because I didn't want your uncle to be left alone, but he wants to live much more than I do.

"I've always wanted to do something special for you. I've never had a child of my own, and I've loved you in my own way. I truly want to help you. Perhaps you will remember me, and that I gave you something when you needed it most."

"It is very good of you to do this. I am very grateful. And of course I shall remember you always."

Aunt Bessie smiles,

"I'm so glad!"

◆   ◆   ◆

Packing one large trunk each, Leola and Demie get all the clothes they need until Christmas into it. All the girls are crying and then laughing while they help the two get ready. They have never been apart before, so they are excited for the two who are going so far from home, but their laughter turns into tears when they realize they won't be seeing them again for months.

Earl helps Uncle Willie get the covered wagon ready to go. They sweep it out then scrub it down because the group will have to sleep in it one night along the way.

They leave early one morning so they can get almost to Statesville to spend the night. Uncle Willie thinks they can then get to Misenheimer the second day. They spread the bedding they bring for their dorm rooms and get a few hours sleep before they are on the road again.

The last words of advice that Uncle Willie gives them:

The Spirit Of God Is Within Each Of Us
Love Thy Neighbor As Thyself
Don't Let The Sun Go Down On Your Wrath
Judge Not!
But The Greatest Gift From God Is Love So Always Say:
I Love You

The lectures are long and tedious, and the bunk beds sag in the middle. They never have enough hot water to take showers, so the water is cold—always cold. More than this, however, is the loneliness of living without their family. When Christmas finally comes, they breathe sighs of relief and head for home when Uncle Willie arrives.

Returning the following year to finish their education, they both secure teaching positions in the northern part of the state. Leola teaches in a small one-room schoolhouse in Iredell County where they have grades one through six. Demie teaches in the same size school about twenty miles away in Yadkin County. She receives a "scrip" for her pay which is good at the grocery store. They promise Leola that she will get paid at the end of the school year if the county has enough money. Meanwhile, each one is living with a different family within the school area for one month each until the year is over.

As her mother before her, Leola has never cut her hair. She spends almost an hour every night brushing it, keeping it clean and shiny, until it is long enough that she can sit on it. Sometimes she lets it flow free so the natural wave can be seen and the curls at the ends stand out. Other times she braids it and winds it round and round her head almost like a hat.

Leola has soft skin with rose cheeks and a red moist mouth. Her eyes, like her mother's, are large and shining and draw the attention of every young man she meets. By the time she is sixteen her breasts are already well developed, and she has small hands and feet. But she is somewhat shy and humble, thinking she is ugly.

Several schools share one principal to visit the schools and give the punishment needed if the female teacher cannot administer it. Within the first year, Demie starts dating her visiting principal, Carlos Privett, but Leola continues to go to cakewalks and socials nearby.

The Beginning Branches

One evening while Leola and Eva are at a cakewalk, Leola looks across the room and sees the handsomest man she has ever seen in her life. She keeps her eye on him as the bidding starts for the cakes. As usual, everybody bids one dollar until she suddenly hears:

"I bid five dollars for the cake that belongs to the most beautiful young lady in the room."

When Leola realizes that he is the one bidding, and he is looking directly at her, she wets her pants.

"How can he possibly think I am beautiful", she thinks, "when I am ugly?"

In a deep voice, he says, "Hi! Yoad. I'm Ray Pharr", and he takes her small hand in his large one.

("Yoad" is the pet name he will call her until the day he dies. No one, not even the kids, will know why)

Not knowing that he is almost a year younger than she, Leola agrees to go out with him. To her surprise, he takes her to see his family. His mother, Martha Goforth Pharr, starts introducing Ray's brothers and sisters to her.

"Ray is the youngest of eleven children. I was forty-eight when he was born," she says; "so many of his nieces and nephews are much older than he. Lydia's daughter Martha is the same age as Ray. She is married to a man named Jeff, so everyone calls them 'Mott and Jeff' as one word. Growing up, Mott and Ray were very close."

Strange, but throughout their married life, Mott and Jeff remain friends along with their son and two daughters. They live in Kannapolis and work in Cannon Mills making towels and bed linen. Ray takes his family to see them at least once a month for the next fifteen years.

Uncle Willie performs the wedding ceremony when Ray and Leola get married the following year. People from Rose Chapel Church bring four wedding cakes, and Aunt Bessie brings one in the shape of a heart. Some say it is the largest wedding of the decade. (No doubt most of it made up of the Pharr clan, for many of the brothers of Ray have nine to eleven children in them).

Ray's family gives them what little money they can spare, and Uncle Willie gives them a cow and some used furniture as a dowry. Ray finds work driving a gasoline truck delivering fuel to the stations throughout the northern part of the county.

Finding a house in the eastern part of Statesville called *Diamond Hill,* Ray and Leola move into it. They can keep a cow and chickens, and they have room for a rather large garden. The house has three bedrooms, a living room with large windows overlooking the front yard, a dining room in combination with the kitchen, and a room just off the hall big enough to store the boxes, trunks, and whatever else of non-immediate use.

Having fallen in love with him, Leola would have followed him wherever he decided they will live, but this house is large enough for a family, and they want a large one.

They awaken at dawn each morning, and while Ray milks the cow, brings it in to strain before putting it into the icebox on the back porch, Leola cooks a breakfast of bacon and eggs because Ray will be driving a big truck and be gone all day.

Not many days pass until she has finished making the curtains, and Ray comes home in time to hang them before supper. She is always looking out the front window, anxiously waiting for him to pull his truck into the driveway and get out to come into the house.

Every time he opens the door and steps down to the ground, Leola shivers with delight. She is somewhat troubled by the beauty and attraction he holds for her. It is more than his physical appearance: a straight, well-cut nose, high light-brown forehead, wavy, glossy, black hair, eyes that are green and rather melancholy at times; five feet eleven inches tall with broad shoulders which he holds erect; muscles in his arms and legs that stand out as he lifts heavy tanks and such in his work.

"How can a handsome man like that love someone like me?" she thinks.

There is tenderness about him as he leads her to the couch after they eat and reaches up to take her hair down. He nightly brushes her hair as he tells her of his day and his thoughts as he goes from station to station.

"I find it hard to believe that a beautiful woman like you with your education can love a guy like me. I've never been to college, and I will never be rich enough to buy you all the things I want you to have. Like my brothers and sisters, I want a large family, and yet I don't know how we can afford them."

"When I was a very young girl, I made a vow to myself that when I grew up and had children, we would never let material things matter. Having two loving parents means more to a child than all the money in the world," answers Leola.

◆   ◆   ◆

Early one morning on November 15th, Lawrence Wesley Pharr arrives at home with a midwife assisting Leola in her own bed. Ray's father, Wesley, died when Ray was quite young, and they want their first son to be named after him. Two years later, on August 22nd, a second son arrives in the same bed with the same midwife assisting. He is named Noah Hillred, after her father Noah. Then two years later, on July 13th, a third son arrives, and they name him Douglas, just Douglas, no middle name, and no one they have known is named Douglas. Two more years, on October 23rd, another son arrives, and they name him George Ray Pharr, Junior.

They want a daughter so much but two years later Leola miscarries, so it is not until another year passes that a daughter arrives on December 7th. They name her Minnie Emily: Minnie is the name of a sister that died and Emily is the name of Leola's grandmother.

To an outsider, the family seems to be "hard up", never very well clothed, and deprived of many comforts and pleasures which seem common enough to others. But Ray and Leola constantly proclaim the love and mercy and care of God for all of them and, of course, teach the children as Uncle Willie taught her:

The Spirit of God Is Within Each Of Us
Love Thy Neighbor As Thyself
Don't Let The Sun Go Down On Your Wrath
Judge Not!
But The Greatest Gift From God Is Love, So Always Say:
I Love You

With so many children, Leola has to have help in keeping the house clean. Ray puts an ad in the paper, and the next day a Black lady from across the railroad tracks over in "Rabbit Town" answers it. Leola hires her to come in during the day Monday through Friday to help with the housework. Her name is Nellie, and she is soon treated as one of the family.

She helps get the work organized by assigning Lawrence to sweep, "Nick", as he likes to be called, to make the beds, Doug to carry out the trash, and Junior to help with the ironing.

Emily loves to sit on her lap, and Ray teases her about it. One day she is sitting on her lap and Ray says:

"Don't you know that by keeping your arm around a Black woman that your arm will turn black?"

Jerking her arm away, she hits the pot bellied stove and burns it. She goes screaming to her mother, and Nellie says:

"Mr. Ray. See what your teasing done?"

After Nellie helps to prepare the meal, she takes her plate and sits at a small table in the kitchen. One day Ray says to her:

"Nellie, if you are good enough to cook it, you can sit with us. Do you think you are better than we are?"

"Oh, no! Mr. Ray. I'm not good enough to eat at the table with white folks."

Ray rearranges the table, and from that day on, Nellie sits at one end of the table and he sits at the other end.

One day Nellie comes in early enough to catch Ray before he goes to work.

"Mr. Ray. My parents want you and your family to come to our house for supper. We're having fried fish."

Soon after they get there, her dad brings out a jug.

"Whisky goes so good with fried fish."

"You go ahead and drink it, but I don't drink. I would love to have a cup of coffee with mine," Ray replies.

Of all the eleven children, Ray's brother, Fred, is the only one who drinks and hunts wild birds and animals. One night he comes to the front door, dead drunk, and Ray goes to the door.

"Sorry, Fred. I can't let you in. No man, brother or not, comes into my home drunk."

When Fred tries to push past him and come in anyway, Ray knocks him out cold. He calls the kids and they drag him into the house. He sleeps it off while lying on the living room floor.

The Roots Sink Deeper

Buying a used Hudson automobile, Ray teaches Leola how to drive. She needs the car to buy groceries and to take the kids to the bus stop when they close Open View Elementary School, and the kids no longer walk to school.

One Sunday Ray has a migraine headache so he stays at home while Leola takes the kids to church. They are members of the Diamond Hill Baptist Church, and the kids haven't missed attending Sunday School for several years. Perfect attendance for seven years has a reward of a new Bible so each kid wants one of his very own.

When the service is over about one o'clock, Leola waits for the parking lot to be empty because she isn't too comfortable in backing a car. Finally, everyone is gone except for Leola and her kids so they get into the car very quietly. Leola takes the crank from under the seat, inserts it at the front of the car and cranks it while the kids watch. She moves it into reverse and puts her foot on the gas pedal. Nerves, excitement, who knows why, but suddenly she mashes down too hard and the car spins round and round in circles, knocking down all the fence posts surrounding the parking lot. The kids begin to scream because they are frightened and don't know what to do.

Getting the car stopped, Leola vows she will never drive a car again. For several years, Ray and the kids beg her to drive, but she refuses to sit behind a steering wheel again.

Come The Depression Years

With a growing family and only one person bringing in any money, Ray and Leola move to the country where the kids can work the land and go to school while Ray continues to drive the truck for an income to live on.

Only ten miles from their old home, they move to a large, two-story house on a farm. There is a front porch running across the entire width of the house with an entrance into a wide hall that has a winding stairway. To the right is the living room with doors opening into the formal dining room. To the left is the den with doors opening into the master bedroom with bath. On down the hall is the door to the kitchen and breakfast room.

There are five bedrooms and bath on the second floor. Having lived all their lives in the city, the kids are frightened when the sun goes down and the house and yard are pitch black. The kerosene lamp in the kitchen makes shadows on the walls, and they have difficulty sleeping for several nights.

Pam and Fanny Morrison, with their adopted daughter, Irene, live on an adjoining farm. Ray and Leola teach the kids:

"Always respect your elders. Use 'Aunt' for a Black lady and 'Uncle' for a Black man. They will call you 'Mister' and 'Miss' along with your first name."

Ray hires Aunt Fanny, as he instructs the kids to call her, to help Leola with the housework, and Uncle Pam to help the boys with the horses and cows. Aunt Fanny is an excellent cook and her pies have the kids begging for seconds. Uncle Pam "roughhouses" with the boys, and they soon climb all over him every time he sits down.

◆   ◆   ◆

Winters can be awfully cold sometimes in North Carolina. People say that every seven years the winters will be more severe than all the other six. Their first winter is one of those seven. It snows for days, and then it sleets on top of that. Weighing over two hundred pounds, Ray walks on top of the snow to the barn to feed the animals.

Locals talk about the year 1927 as being the worst they can remember. They are so thankful when spring finally comes even though it means the farm work will begin. Not many men remember those days before all the new fangled equipment was developed.

Most farm boys don't begin school until they're six or seven. They are usually needed on the farm. Junior begs his mother to teach him to read at an early age so when he is five, she says that he should be in school and out from underfoot.

The local school is made up of farm kids, so the school board arranges the school calendar whereby there is a Fall Break for gathering the farm crops and a Spring Break for planting them.

By Spring Break, the snow melts and the ground thaws. Uncle Pam helps Lawrence and Nick get the horses harnessed and hitched to the plow. They go out into the fields and break up the ground for planting. Doug and Junior drop the seeds of corn one by one in the rows and then cover them up. By mid-morning, Leola has finished the breakfast dishes and started the noonday meal. When Aunt Fanny arrives, Leola comes to the field and helps with the covering until a little before lunchtime, then she returns to the house.

By six o'clock everyone is tired and hungry, but they each have chores to do before they eat. Leola finishes cooking the evening meal and Aunt Fanny goes home to cook theirs. Lawrence and Nick take care of the horses by taking them down to the branch to drink. Then taking off their harness, they put them into their stalls to eat. Doug and Junior feed the pigs and chickens, and Junior gathers the eggs. After each one has milked his cow, they go into the house and get cleaned up for supper.

Ray is way before his time in his respect and treatment of women and the way he helps around the house. When he comes home from work, he quickly washes his hands and helps Leola prepare the meal. She usually asks him to make the homemade biscuits for she says his come out soft and fluffy and hers don't always turn out that way.

When he's not working on Saturday, he wakes all the kids with,

"Shhh. Don't wake your mother. She has worked hard all week and needs to sleep in this morning."

Not before they sweep floors, dust, gather the laundry, and help their dad with breakfast (usually ham and eggs with toast) do they wake their mother, and she acts so surprised each time.

◆   ◆   ◆

Living on a farm in the nineteen twenties without machinery requires long hours and hard work, but Ray and Leola grew up on a farm, and they know what must be done. These are the depression years since the stock market crashed and many people commit suicide, and millions are out of work.

Leola knows the value of food as well as money, but she also knows the likes and dislikes of each of her children. Cooking the meals is somewhat like cooking for a restaurant because she tries to please the taste of each one. Junior doesn't like any kind of sauce or mustard on a sandwich; Douglas does. Junior doesn't drink milk, so Douglas drinks his milk when no one is looking, and they exchange glasses. Lawrence won't drink anything, not even medicine, if he knows it has alcohol in it; he refuses to taste it. Nick is the only one who likes chicken livers; he always eats all of them whenever they have chicken for dinner. Emily likes most anything to eat, but she is really hard to please in what clothes she wears.

With four boys so close in age, all the clothes, except shoes, are passed down until they wear out. Poor Junior never gets anything new because he wears what Lawrence passes down to Nick, Nick to Doug, Doug to Junior. He wails when their dad buys Nick and Doug identical beige suits for them to wear to their prom. Now he will be forced to wear the same color to his prom as well as every event that calls for a suit.

◆   ◆   ◆

But it's not all work and no play. Every day when Ray comes home from work, all the kids drop everything and rush to sit on his lap. Without fail, he has a small brown bag of penny candy to give each kid, but the nickel piece is saved for Leola.

"Wait! Wait! Whoever loves me the most gets the biggest piece. Let's start with the youngest. Emily, spread your hands as far as your love for me can reach."

Of course each piece is about the same, but the kids take turns seeing how far their arms can reach. Each one takes his candy, hugs and kisses him, and says, "I love you, daddy."

Occasionally, on a Saturday, they drive into town to watch a motion picture show. There is the *Crescent* that shows cowboy shows with stars like Bob Steele, Ken Maynard, Tom Mix and others, but these are their favorites. *The Playhouse* shows serious things about politics and such, but Leola is the only one interested in that kind, and they seldom go there. Then they build *The State* that shows pictures about love and romance that aren't very interesting to any of them.

Very early on Saturdays the boys gather wood and build a fire under the wash pot out in the backyard while their mother scrubs the clothes by hand on a washboard and then puts the white ones into the pot to boil.

After taking them from the pot, she hangs them on the clothesline to dry in the sun, leaving them clean and white as snow.

That night, she stays up late to dampen them down, wait for the iron to heat on the back of the stove, and then irons them before midnight.

Knowing how Ray loves the smoothness, Leola irons the sheets to go on their bed, his white shorts to be near his skin, and the clothes the kids will be wearing tomorrow morning.

Every Sunday Leola dresses all the boys in white pants and white shirts and Emily in a white dress. They arrive at New Hope Baptist Church for Sunday School at 9:30 AM and then Preaching at 11. If the preacher is long winded and goes past noon, the kids get restless. Even some of the parents start squirming in the pews because nobody wants to wait past one for dinner. (Dinner is the meal in the middle of the day and Supper is the evening meal.) Sunday afternoons just fly for they are back at church by seven for BYPU (Baptist Young People's Union) and Preaching again at eight.

When the weather is nice and warm and no danger of snow in the mountains, sometimes they rush home from church and grab the picnic basket they prepared earlier in the day and drive to the Blue Ridge Mountains. Leola points out the breathtaking beauty of all the wild flowers and the different colors of the leaves on the trees. At Blowing Rock, they gaze in wonder at the scenery, and she reminds them:

"God provides all this for our pleasure so remember in your prayers tonight to thank Him for it."

In the heat of the summer when the kids get restless on a Sunday afternoon, Ray and Leola take them to the bottomland where the South Yadkin River runs by. No one else lives for miles around so they take off their clothes and go wading or swimming in the river. The three older boys learn to swim in that river, but Junior isn't quite ready for it just yet.

One summer during the revival meetings, Rev. McSwain listens to the Pharr boys singing and asks them to sing a hymn by themselves. They shake their heads and smile. When he asks Junior if he will stand in a chair and sing a solo, his parents smile with pride when he sings two stanzas from Amazing Grace.

Until his voice begins to crackle and change, Junior sings during the service every summer, standing in a chair so everyone can see him from the back of the church.

◆   ◆   ◆

One day when the boys are hoeing corn in the bottomland and the weather is extremely hot, they take off their clothes and go into the river to cool off. As they climb out of the river, they find wild blackberries on the banks and pick them to eat. That night they begin to itch and burn but can't find any reason for it. Suddenly, Junior yells out:

"Daddy! Daddy! Come quick! I think we have scarlet fever!"

When Ray opens their door, he bursts out laughing.

"You kids must have been picking blackberries today. You have chiggers. Let's go downstairs, and I'll wipe kerosene on you. They will die and you won't itch anymore."

Now that they know about chiggers, they are very careful when they pick wild berries for their mother to can. During the summers, Leola cans beans, corn, tomatoes, berries, and most anything that can be put into a jar. Ray robs the beehives so she uses honey to sweeten the berries to save on sugar.

◆   ◆   ◆

Ray's mother, Martha, (Granny to the kids), and his sister, Callie Mae, (Aunt Cal), live on a small farm in the northern part of the county. Aunt Cal is a large woman, never been married, so she works the farm while Granny cooks the meals, washes their clothes, and cleans the house. Junior is the only kid who spends a few weeks each summer with them.

Aunt Cal builds a pond for him in the branch that flows by their house. She sits on the banks and watches him as he catches small fish and puts them into little ponds he has made. At the end of the day, she tears down the mud that she used to hold the water, and the fish swim down the stream.

Some days she takes him fishing with her as they sit for hours on the banks. He always squeals with delight when she catches a big one for he knows she will clean it for their supper that night.

When they need it, Aunt Cal gathers the eggs, puts them into a basket that Granny has woven, and she and Junior walk to the little country store about two miles away. After she has exchanged the eggs for snuff, sugar, and coffee, she lifts him high enough to look into the candy showcase, and he points to the ones he wants.

When his parents arrive to pick him up, Junior begs to stay longer, but it is time for him to get home so they can buy school supplies and get ready for another school year.

Love Thy Neighbor As Thyself

Farmers make good neighbors. In the fall when the crops are ready to be harvested, each family picks its own cotton and pulls its own corn. The shucking of corn is just too long and boresome to do alone, so each family pulls the corn and piles it high in the barnyard. The stalks are tied in bundles to be fed to the cows and horses during the winter. Taking turns, each farmer asks his wife to make pies and cakes and lots of cookies; then they invite all the neighbors to come over one night, usually Saturday, for a "corn shucking".

They bring all their kids who get together to make ice cream to go with the cakes and pies, and they squeeze lemons to make lemonade. Out in the barnyard the men and women begin to sing, usually hymns, and the kids take them lemonade and push the shucks back so they can continue with their shucking and not have to get up.

Long about nine o'clock, they take a break to eat the goodies and chat for a little while. Soon, all the small kids crawl into the soft shucks and fall asleep. Finished or not with the shucking, at midnight, the adults hold hands in a circle and say a prayer before going home for the night.

◆   ◆   ◆

A portion of each evening is set aside for reading the Bible and listening to one in the group who will explain some of it to the others. Each kid takes his turn studying the scripture so he can explain it. When the readers get stumped, their mother explains it for them.

Leola explains most things to the kids, especially when have a question about sex.

"Your father was born when his mother was forty-eight years old, and there was no one left to talk with him about sex. It embarrasses him when one of you kids asks him anything about it, so you feel free to ask me. I don't want you kids picking up things from other kids. They might give you the wrong information."

She is always glad to answer their questions, but it makes her sad when she has to punish one of them. As a teacher, she always left the extreme punishment of her students to the visiting principal. With their children, she and Ray had agreed that she must punish them part of the time so they wouldn't associate him with it.

For minor infractions, she has each kid cut a small hickory limb so she can switch just the legs. As she switches, she begins to cry and beg them to quit doing whatever they have done because it hurts her too much to punish them. They begin to cry when she begins:

"You know this is hurting me much more than it hurts you. We only want for you to have roots that are grounded in love and family so you can soar like an eagle all your life and know you will land safely."

◆   ◆   ◆

Aunt Cal's back starts giving her a lot of trouble, and she has difficulty in running their small farm. Leola begs Ray to ask his sister and mother to move in with them.

"We have plenty of room. Remember my early childhood? It will be wonderful for the children to have so many family members to surround them with love."

Unfortunately, Granny gets sick a few months after they move in and is too weak to climb the stairs to their room. Ray buys a hospital bed and moves her down to the living room. Now it's easy for everyone to check on her whenever she calls out. Soon her coughing and loud breathing is heard throughout the house, but during the night it keeps bothering them when they try to sleep.

1930's

Two More Branches

On April 17th, Ray jumps into the truck and brings Aunt Fanny to the house to help Leola when Hugh Gilbert Pharr arrives, a seven pound five ounce baby boy. Now the house is filled with Granny's coughing and wheezing and Hugh Gilbert crying during the night. He is only ten days old when Granny dies in her sleep one night.

After the funeral, the family gathers in the living room so their parents can talk with them about Granny and about death. Ray begins with:

"Now, kids. My mother's dying is sad, and we will all miss her, but it is not a tragedy. She lived a good, rewarding life and saw her kids, grandkids, and even great grandkids grow and become good people. God called her home where she will never have any more pain or trouble breathing, so we must be happy for her. It's ok if you want to go to your rooms and cry for awhile, but please don't think there is anything wrong in her dying."

"If having your granny die isn't a tragedy, then what is, for gosh sakes," cries Junior as he puts his head into his mother's lap.

During her seventh month of pregnancy, Leola has difficulty keeping up with the housework and working in the fields so Ray hires Irene to come to the house each day with Aunt Fanny. She takes over the responsibility of looking after Hugh Gilbert, who is cross and cranky cutting teeth, and often chews and slobbers on Irene's arm. When Aunt Fanny sees that this is going on, she immediately says:

"Irene! Don't let that white child chew on your black arm. Shame on you! You know better than that!"

Dr. Sharpe drives out from Statesville on April 10th to assist Leola in the birth of Robert Reece Pharr. As he is leaving, he talks with Hugh Gilbert and asks him his name.

"My name is Bill Hoover," is the answer he gets. No one will ever know why the child said such a thing, but from then on, everyone calls him "Billy". Later, when he goes to school, he tells his teacher that his name is

Billy. Leola finds that all his school records list him as Billy, and since Billy doesn't like the name of Hugh, she takes him to the courthouse and officially changes his name to William Gilbert Pharr.

◆   ◆   ◆

Sliding down the banisters, Nick falls and breaks his arm. Ray rushes him to the hospital where they put it in a sling. Suddenly, he is a hero because no one in the family has ever been in a hospital. He struts around the house for days, proclaiming:

"I don't have to go to sccchhhhool. I don't have to go to sccchhhhol."

Lawrence and Douglas envy him, but Junior loves school and stays up later every night in order to be prepared for each day's work. At the end of the school year, he gets all 'A's while the others get 'A's and 'B's, and Nick is held back because he missed so much school. Now he tells everybody:

"Because of a tragedy, I am repeating a grade in school."

The family knows it wasn't a tragedy, but they agree it is a real tragedy when Ray is brought home one evening in shock. While driving his truck out on Chipley Ford Road, a little boy only six years old runs out in front of him and gets killed. Leola immediately puts him to bed and crawls in with him. The kids hear him sobbing way into the night.

From that day on, he refuses to drive a large truck or to go out that road again. He finds a job selling furniture and works inside for years.

Limbs Reach Out

As the older children reach their teenage years, their individual lives take shape rather early. Although Lawrence is named after his grandfather Wesley on his father's side, he looks, acts, and thinks like his Uncle Willie on his mother's side. He is serious about life and accepts his responsibilities when left in charge when their parents leave them alone. When Nick and Doug get into a fight, he steps in to stop them. They usually accept it and stop immediately.

The kids seldom snitch on each other so nothing is said when their parents return home, but it is evident they are angry over something. Bedtime arrives, but before they are excused to go to their rooms, Leola calls them aside.

"You two know you cannot go to bed with anger between you. Talk it through so you can go to bed in peace. The sun must never set with anger in the home. Don't forget to say I Love You".

Nick looks, acts, and thinks like his Uncle Earl, although he is named after his grandfather Noah. He has a way about the way he talks and acts toward children that makes the younger ones look up to him. He can be very serious about his duties of looking after the young ones, but he has a lighter side that Lawrence doesn't seem to have. He teases them and the twinkle in his eyes betrays him.

Nothing like the other two in looks, acts, or thinking, Doug is full of mischief and somewhat lazy. Well, lazy about carrying about his responsibilities, but full of energy in figuring out ways to get out of any kind of physical work. He spends more time in getting out of doing a particular chore than it would take him to do the actual chore.

He teases everyone, including his mother and dad. When his mother asks him to get a switch so she can switch his legs, he breaks it at just the right places so it wraps around his legs and doesn't hurt very much. When she says:

"This is going to hurt me much more than it does you."

Then he says:

"Then switch your legs instead of mine."

She usually gets so tickled that she laughs and forgets to punish him.

The only girl among six boys, Emily doesn't become "spoiled" as many a girl might be. She is healthy and playful and loves to sit on her daddy's feet. She puts her arms around his legs and begs him to swing her back and forth until his legs ache, and he has to take her off his legs and hold her on his lap.

He is the only one who can cut her hair, so he cuts it the same way every time: in a bob somewhat like Little Orphan Annie from the comics. When she tattle-tells on Doug, he knows she doesn't like to be called Minnie, so he whispers to her for days:

"Minnie Emily, Minnie Emily, the little girl with the Orphan Annie haircut."

◆   ◆   ◆

Reaching the teens, Junior decides he wants to be called Ray J., so everyone tries to remember to call him that. Everyone, that is, except Doug. He teases and calls him "Dunnie" because he knows it makes him angry.

Ray J. has the looks of his dad, but loves to read and takes after his mother in doing the laundry and helping her in the kitchen, obviously a teacher in the making.

One by one, each boy sits on his dad's lap and learns to drive a car. At sixteen, Nick takes the test and gets a job driving the bus back and forth to school. With school twenty-two miles away, everyone has to get up an hour earlier. They know he will go off and leave them if they aren't ready on time. They beg him to quit the job, but once a Pharr gives his word, nothing is going to make him break it. Their parents teach them:

"A man's word is as good as his bond."

During the dead of winter it gets dark by the time they get home from school, but they still have to milk the cows, feed the horses, hogs, and chickens before they come in to eat. Ray J. is the last one in because he gathers the eggs and sometimes has to crawl under the smokehouse to get those where the hens have stolen their nests. His mother cautions him:

"You be careful crawling under there after dark. Snakes or other animals could be under there and bite you."

To Ray J. it seems school barely gets started in the fall, and then it's cotton picking time. School lets out for "Fall Break" which is really time out from school so the farmers' kids can pick cotton and gather the crops. Most kids don't enjoy school the way Ray J. does so they look forward to staying home, but he complains about having a backache every day from dragging his toe sack and picking cotton so close to the ground. His dad teases him:

"There's no way you can have a backache. Everybody knows that people don't have spines until they're twenty-one years old."

By daybreak each day, Aunt Cal goes to the fields with them to pick cotton. Doug rushes down the row and then sits in the shade, waiting for them to catch up. Ever so often, Aunt Cal, who comes behind him in the row next to him so she can check up on him, hollers across the field:

"Douglas Pharr. You come back here right this minute. Quit leaving so much in the burrs; that's wasteful! Waste not! Want not!"

When they get to the house, Doug complains to his mother:

"Aunt Cal is an old maid and bosses us around."

"Young man. I could very easily have been an old maid if I had not met your father, and then you wouldn't be here. You should be thankful your aunt is out there working like a dog to help us finish picking the cotton before winter sets it. Go tell your aunt how much you love her."

When they load the cotton in the wagon and take it to the cottongin, they pack it into bales. Pure white cotton brings the most money so they are careful not to have burrs or trash in their bags. Their dad uses the money from cotton to buy the seed and fertilizer for the next spring planting as well as for sugar and coffee and things in general for the house.

Fall is the time for Uncle Fred to come visit because he knows how to sugar-cure ham. They raise hogs for the ham, sausage, and lard they need for the winter months. They also raise cows for most of the meat they eat is beef. Every winter the smokehouse is full of meat. They wrap it in brown paper and put it into sacks to be hung from the rafters so the air will keep it from spoiling.

◆   ◆   ◆

When Ray J. graduates from high school at age sixteen, he goes to Mitchell College. It is close and not too expensive. He takes a part time job working as a drug store cowboy serving mostly cokes and icecream. It doesn't pay very well, but he doesn't need very much.

When Nick and Doug graduate, they find jobs at Cannon Mills in Kannapolis working on the night shift. Everyone wonders why Doug ever thought he could work during those hours. He quits after two weeks and comes home to work during the day. Those nights are the time for living, if you are Doug. Selling furniture from nine to five is more his style.

Barely eighteen years old, Lawrence is sometimes thought to be Ray's brother—he acts so old. He is tall, with brown hair, already wearing glasses, and a serious look, sometimes even a frown, on his face. He marries Mildred Smith, his girlfriend since the 10th grade in school.

Mildred is the daughter of George and Rosie Smith, who own the adjoining farm and attend the same church, New Hope Baptist. She has red hair, cut very short, somewhat like a boy's, with freckles on her upturned nose and dancing green eyes. In outward appearance, she is the opposite from Lawrence—laughing and teasing and fun to be around.

There is a small house across the road from the family. Lawrence and Mildred move in, buy a bed, a couch, two chairs, and a refrigerator to finish out the furnishings of the house. For the first time, they have the thrill of possession. They are so excited that the first night they go to bed in their new home they lie awake talking until four o'clock in the morning.

Their son, Lawrence, Jr., is born just two years after Bob is born. Then two years later they have a daughter named Velma Jean.

Ray often teases Lawrence by saying he got married when he was eighteen and on his next birthday he turned fifty-one. Lawrence does seem old for his age. He is always so serious minded and should have been a preacher like his Uncle Willie for he lives and breathes by the Bible.

He sometimes has a few light moments when he teases Mildred.

"You know that in the beginning when God created man, he named him Pharr. Every time a man becomes sinful, God changes his name so that is the reason there are so few men left named Pharr."

Two years after moving to Kannapolis, Nick meets Winnifred Childers, a woman who runs the machine next to his. Winnie is an attractive woman with brown hair that is always perfectly groomed (she goes to the beauty salon every Friday), and a smile and quick wit about her. They take their short breaks together and chat about their personal lives. Nick tells her that he hasn't met any nice girls to date, and she tells him that she is married.

She is a year older than he and about two inches taller. He seems like a nice gentleman, so she confides in him about her abusive husband.

"Some nights he is already drunk when I leave for work. I dread going home to him. I hope and pray he is asleep when I get there."

The following year, telling only Doug about her past, Nick brings her home to meet his parents and announces they are married.

Doug meets Helen Gomerry, who works at Lazenby Jewelry Store and lives on Davie Avenue, walking distance from where he lives. She is tall and thin with black hair and blue eyes, somewhat reserved, which is something new for him.

Doug is the handsome son who takes after his dad in looks: tall, with broad shoulders that he holds erect in order to show off his slim waist. He has blonde hair with a natural wave in it but the same green eyes of his dad that seem to dance when he flirts with a young girl. He has always dated the bubbly, outgoing young girls who are obviously out for a good time. His mother often questions his motives when he has dated certain girls.

But Helen has an attraction for him that no other girl has had. She has a younger sister, Winifred, and Doug arranges a double date with Ray J. and Winnie to attend the late night movie on Saturday night at 10:30. The four of them enjoy it so much that it becomes a regular for them every Saturday night for over a year.

The movie ends promptly at twelve o'clock. There are "blue laws" that forbid any business to operate between the hours of twelve midnight on Saturday until 6 AM on Monday morning. The four them go back to Mrs. Gomerry's house until about two o'clock or later. Ray J. and Winnie are always involved in reading some romantic novel in a book or magazine, but Doug and Helen often slip downstairs to the basement.

Everyone is surprised when Helen agrees to marry Doug, and even more surprised when they move into the house with Helen's family. The house is large enough, but a young married couple living with that many people in the house causes some eyebrows to raise. Only Ray J. knows the real reason they get married because Doug told him long ago that Helen excites him more than any other girl he has ever known.

1940's

Testing the Tree

Suddenly, the Japanese bomb Pearl Harbor, on December 7th, Emily's birthday. That event marks the day their lives will be changed forever. Hoyle Smith, Mildred's oldest brother, is a sailor. Word came right away that he was killed aboard his ship at Pearl. He had married some girl from Oregon. None of the family ever got to see her since she never came to North Carolina.

Lawrence is turned down for the service because his health isn't good. Besides, he is married, and they have two kids. Nick joins the Army and goes into basic training. Doug thinks the Marines are more exciting, so he joins and leaves town the next month.

Ray J. wants to join the Marines and be near Doug. But they tell him that since he qualifies for the Navy and they need men in the Navy right now that he should go there. He winds up in boot camp near Baltimore, Maryland.

He has never been away from home before and that seems a long way for him. Most of the guys moan and groan about having to get up at six in the morning, but he has no trouble with that since he has spent his whole life getting up at five. He does have trouble with taking showers with about fifty strangers at one time. Sleeping on a cot in the barracks with at least a hundred or more takes some getting used to.

As each son leaves for his tour of service, the whole family gathers at the bus or train depot to see the departure. The younger kids hug and tell each one "I love you", and then their mother does same, trying very hard to hold back the tears. Their dad is the last to give each one a bear hug and a kiss on the cheek.

Winnie moves in with her mother while Nick is in basic training. He comes home for a short furlough and then goes to Camp Robinson in Missouri. Winnie quits her job and goes to be with him. Staying there for only a few weeks, his next stop is in Colorado Springs, Colorado. Winnie, of course, goes with him, and finds a small apartment in somebody's attic where they live for three months before he goes to Europe to serve in the ambulance corps.

Doug's wife, Helen, lives with her mother, two sisters, and two brothers. When she gets word that Doug has been injured while out on the desert in training, the family wonders why she doesn't go to him, but she refuses to leave her mother and family.

Ray J. comes home and announces that he has decided to take the training to become a bomb disposal expert. His mother starts crying because it sounds so dangerous, and his dad says:

"Son, I thought you were a pretty smart kid, but you don't know 'cum here from sic um."

They feel much better about it when he is sent to Washington, D.C. and comes home every other weekend on the train. He explains that it will not be too dangerous if he studies hard and learns how to do his job properly.

Bomb Disposal

The WAVES have overtaken the campus of the American University in Washington, D.C. (Women Accepted for Volunteer Emergency Service.) There are thousands and thousands of them in the mess hall where the few navy men have to eat.

The classes are small, only about twenty when they start, but more than half of them flunk out the first week. Classes start each morning at eight o'clock. They have thirty minutes for lunch, and then it is back to class, listening, taking notes, watching film, and trying to understand what each instructor is telling about bombs, fuzes, missiles, projectiles, and a little about mines, until 6 o'clock. Each instructor warns them every hour to listen and ask questions. They will be tested each Friday on what is covered for the week, but, most importantly, for the few who finish the course, their lives will depend on how well they do when they work on a live bomb later.

During their weeks of training, they have their weekends free. It's almost like going to regular school and not being in service at all. Two other guys, George and Tiny, and Ray J. live in a house not very far from the University, and George has a car. George starts dating a WAVE named Barbara and pretty soon gets so love sick that they are disgusted with him.

George has a drinking problem, and whenever Barbara won't or can't go out with him, he goes to a bar and gets drunk. The first night he did that, Ray J. is home alone studying when he comes in. He doesn't exactly come in quietly; he bangs on the door and startles Ray J. almost out of his wits—his first time to be that up close to someone who is drunk. George runs to the bathroom, vomiting, and yells for someone to bring a wet washcloth. Then he starts crying,

"Barbara doesn't love me. I know it. Why doesn't Barbara love me? I love her. Tell me, why doesn't Barbara love me? I love Barbara."

Tiny comes in about that time, so between them, they get him undressed and to bed. Tiny says,

"This isn't the first time this has happened. It's nothing serious. He won't remember a thing about it in the morning."

While Tiny goes home to Boston nearly every weekend, Ray J. catches the train every other weekend to go down home. He meets a student nurse named Marilee, and soon they are getting pretty serious about each other. Marilee is in her second year of training with only one year to go before she takes the final examination to become a registered nurse. She is somewhat of a tomboy with freckles on her nose, brown hair, slender, quite pretty, but seems shy when he brings her home to meet his parents. She shudders when they hug her and announces that she doesn't like to be hugged and kissed.

Now Ray J. comes home to see her, and they seldom have time to talk with anyone but themselves. One weekend they slip across the state line and get married by the justice of the peace in South Carolina. They don't sleep together for four months until Marilee and Emily come to Washington, D. C., for two weeks' vacation.

After Ray J. takes his final exam, he goes to the Navy Department where they explain the procedures necessary for him to have access to classified material that he will be using in working on bombs and missiles. The group has been told they have been carefully investigated since they will be reading highly classified and sometimes secret materials.

The group has ten days delayed orders to report to Oakland, California, where they will board a transport ship to the South Pacific. One of the instructors tells Ray J. he can bum an airplane ride out to San Diego free of charge. They are taking fighter planes out there. He can hardly believe it, since Doug is stationed there in a hospital as a corpsman. He had gotten injured in training and couldn't continue with his original plans. The pilot settles Ray J. into the radioman's position and they take off for San Diego. Every time they come to a large city or place of interest, he flies low and tells Ray J. what each one is (Ray J. had told him he had never been out west).

Ray J. makes a huge mistake when they land for refueling at Fort Worth, Texas, and he drinks a large chocolate milkshake. They barely get into the air before the wind starts blowing and the plane is wobbling from side to side and up and down and that milkshake starts doing the same thing. He is really glad to get there and get out of that plane.

What a great time Doug and Ray. J. have during the remainder of his time before reporting to Oakland! They try to get caught up on every member of the family. It has been some time since Doug has been home so there is much to be said. Finally, he says,

"Why haven't you mentioned getting married? In your letters you haven't said anything either. I thought you and I never kept secrets from each other?"

"Well, I'm not real proud of the way I rushed into that without some advice from you or Nick. I don't really know that much about her, and we only had one weekend together. The less said, the better, I guess."

He changes the subject and starts talking about their Mother and Dad. Without many days left, the subject of marriage doesn't come up again, which is a relief.

The experience in Oakland is one for the books. Some time before, the Japanese people who had been rounded up and taken from their homes were first housed in the former racetrack. The Red Cross had intervened and said it wasn't fit for them to live there. They don't object when the navy personnel are housed in the same stalls. This is where they live until they board ship.

They had put two sets of bunks into each stall, one set on each side of the door. Four sailors are in each stall. Crowded, but it has its funny moments. Every morning about sunup, several guys from the Midwest open up the top part of the door, stick their heads over the lower part and bray just like a jackass. Most of the guys don't find it funny at all and throw shoes at them. After a few days, everyone expects it and then they all have a great laugh about it.

Seventeen Days at Sea

The bomb disposal unit is one of four that are Mobil Explosive Investigative Units, better known as MEIU. There are twenty bomb disposal experts in each with seamen attached who will dig out the bombs and missiles. Their small unit could have gotten lost aboard the ship that has over three thousand men aboard if they hadn't assigned quarters close together.

The first few days aboard the huge ship are exciting because none of them had ever been on a ship before. They told them beforehand never to call it a boat, or everyone would know they were landlovers.

Some of the guys admit they are uneasy during a storm so they go below deck. Ray J. loves a storm. He stays on top deck and watches as the waves begin to build high and the thunder gets louder and louder and the lightening starts out in the distance and gradually comes closer until it comes down and dances across the water, throwing sparks like Christmas sparklers. The beauty and wonders that God created makes him want to cry.

He gets a little nervous when the ship goes almost straight up into the air when a big wave comes, and then it pops when it hits the water coming down. In his prayers that night he thanks God for the calm that came after the storm.

Two nights later it is a different storm that comes when planes come out of nowhere and the night lights up with bombs bursting and missiles flying. Men are running in all directions with nowhere to go. They are on a transport ship and carry no guns. All they can do is go below deck and climb into their hammocks and pray. Ray J. includes in his prayers a special one for his parents. He knows they are worse off than he because they have no idea of where he is, where he is going, and when and if he will ever return.

When they hear the all clear sound, everybody hollers and screams, and no one is ashamed to admit he has been afraid. The Captain comes on the loudspeaker and tells them,

"Our sister ship has been hit and we are taking on their three thousand men. The days ahead are going to be rough. Food will have to be cut back, extra hammocks must be strung up, and no one will be allowed above deck after dark without a special pass."

They find out some of the difficulties immediately. Now they are sleeping six decks below and seven hammocks high. Furthermore, now they have an apple, orange, banana, or some other fruit midmorning, and then one hot meal mid-afternoon.

To be down that low and with so many guys crowded together, sleep is almost impossible. Ray J. lucks out when he gets a top hammock. It gets him out of having guys upchuck during the night and it coming down on top of him while he sleeps. One poor guy on the fourth hammock jumps out of bed and lands in a pile of vomit that makes everyone sick.

South Pacific—Not the Musical

Seventeen days of this life is enough to make the war seem far away. When they sight land, the shouts of six thousand guys are enough to wake the devil.

Every time there is a bomb or missile of any kind that lands in the South Pacific and it doesn't go off, their unit is called upon to dismantle it. They go out by ship or plane, depending on where they need them.

Each time a unit goes out on call, all the guys gather round and say goodbye. During the early ones, they are nervous and on edge until they return. They know what is possible each trip. As they get more and more calls and no one gets hurt, they begin to be more casual and assume every-one will return.

The unit gets a cable from the Navy Department that the Italians have found out what they are doing and have come up with a buzz bomb that deliberately will not explode when it lands. They have put a fuze in it that will explode if anyone tries to take it out. Pretty soon the other countries do the same.

They call all the units back to the homebase to study the new methods they receive. Now, when they go out, in addition to the normal tools, they take chemicals with them. They are to mix them and inject the fuze to freeze the pin. This way it won't go off and detonate the bomb. Once again, they gather round the team as they leave on an assignment and worry until they return.

A Kidney, not Rolling, Stone

One Saturday morning, Ray J. rushes to the head, which is his usual habit. Try as he might, nothing comes out, and he feels like he can't wait any longer or he will explode. All day long, he is in and out of the head and gets absolutely no results. He trys to sleep when night comes, thinking if he can relax then he can go. He gets so miserable he finds the corpsman.

"It's a blockage somewhere between the bladder and the end of your penis. Come on back to the cot. I can at least put a hot water bottle on your stomach."

They fly a doctor in from another island, and he says he is passing a kidney stone. He just has to wait for the urine to push it on out. They give him some morphine, so he thinks he can handle it. By afternoon the morphine doesn't do any good, and he is beginning to do more than moan; he is screaming. The doctor says he can see something in the passageway, but it isn't moving. He calls four seamen in and says,

"One guy on each limb and hold this guy down. I'm going in."

In the meantime, it takes weeks for the mail to catch up with them, and Marilee is two months pregnant by the time Ray J. hears about it. Imagine that, Ray J., a father! That couldn't be. He's not ready to settle down and get a job and support a family. He hasn't lived yet.

For months they hover around when Ray J. gets mail. He gets a delayed cable saying he is the father of a beautiful baby daughter. Now the guys begin to call him "daddy", and he's the youngest guy in the outfit.

Before too long, they feel like a big family for everyone talks a lot once they get relaxed. Then, too, when a person's very life depends on other guys doing their part, they become like brothers. It becomes natural to put an arm around a guy when he gets a "Dear John" letter from home or is upset about something.

North Carolina

Three years younger than Ray J., Emily has teachers who keep reminding her that they have had all brothers before her, so they know all the tricks of the family in trying to get out of schoolwork. They keep calling her "Pharr" as if she doesn't have a first name, so she quits answering the roll until they call "Emily".

Luckily for her, Ray buys a furniture store called *Railroad Salvage,* and the family moves back into town. Emily is happy to get into a different school as well as get away from living on a farm. The store is small, located near the depot on South Center Street, so Ray and Lawrence don't need any help in running it. The previous owner had run away with a young high school girl, leaving his wife and four daughters.

For the first time, the family lives in a brick home out on Highway 10 on the west side of town, called *Woodlawn.* Emily attends one school and Bill and Bob attend another. At last, Emily is on her own to make friends who have no connection with her older brothers. By the time she is sixteen years old, Emily is a beautiful young lady with thick, curly hair, creamy complexioned, tiny waist, full bosomed, and a smile that turns the head of all the customers in the restaurant where she works part-time.

Ray and Leola are concerned when she starts dating an older, worldlier man, who is on the Class D baseball team that has recently settled in Statesville. When purchasing a box seat just above third base, Ray never dreams that she would take an interest in one of the players, but they are relieved when she shows an interest in a local boy named Vince who had been in her class at school.

Frank Arey returns from the Merchant Marines on a ten-day leave, stops in at Troutman's Restaurant for a piece of pie and a cup of coffee. He sits down at the counter and waits for Emily to serve him, but she is too busy talking to a young man. He calls to her, but she takes no notice. He calls again and raps the counter.

"How do you do," he says.

"You seem to be in a big hurry," she looks at him with an insolent manner.

"I say. What is the matter with you?" He asks.

"If you will kindly give me your order, I will get what you want. I can't stand here talking all night."

"Apple pie and coffee, please," Frank answers briefly.

He is furious with her. He has a newspaper with him and reads it elaborately until she brings his order.

"If you will give me my bill now, I won't trouble you again," he says icily.

She writes out the slip, places it on the counter in front of him, and goes back to chatting with the young man. Now she is talking to him with animation. Frank decides he will never come to this restaurant again.

But the snub the waitress inflicts on him stays on his mind. If she had been civil to him, he would have been indifferent to her, but now his pride is wounded. He cannot suppress a desire to get even with her.

The next day he goes to the restaurant which he had vowed he would not do. He sees the waitress the moment he comes in so he sits down at one of her tables. He expects her to make some reference to the night before; but when Emily comes to take his order, she says nothing. She gives no sign that she has ever seen him before, so he places his order and waits for her return.

"I say," he says suddenly. "There is a musical comedy playing at the State Theatre. Would you go with me one night to see it?"

"I get off early on Thursday," she replies.

Emily wears a long cloak of some rough, dark material and a shawl over her head. They reach the theatre and find their seats. She gives him a smile and says, "I've never been here before."

Removing her cloak, he sees she is wearing a pale blue dress, cut square at the neck, and her hair is more elaborately arranged.

"I was surprised when you asked me to the theatre", she says, and then doesn't say a word until the movie is over.

He thinks that the next day she will tell everyone at work that he had taken her out and bored her to death. On the way to her house he asks,

"Will you come out with me again one evening?"

Limbs Spring Back

That summer, the U.S. drops the atom bomb and the war ends soon after. The entire family is at the depot when Ray J. gets off the train, but he has some trouble finding them. A bunch of servicemen come home that day. It looks like most of the town is here.

His Mom and Dad have aged a little, but Marilee has changed so much he barely recognizes her. Her hair is long, and she has gained quite a bit since he has seen her. But, the biggest surprise is seeing Anne for the first time. Marilee is holding her when he sees them. She puts her down, and she walks toward him with her arms outstretched (Marilee tells him later how they used his pictures and taught her to know him). Can you imagine seeing your daughter for the first time and she is walking? He sits down on the ground and holds her hand. He tells her that he is her daddy, and he loves her very much. It takes several days for her to warm up to him, but he knows to go slow in working with kids.

Everyone tells him how much he has changed since he left home—that he looks so much older and no longer a boy. If they knew what he'd been through, they would understand. Someone once wrote that war says to youth:

"Send me a boy and I will send home a man."

That is evident in the Pharr family. Although Nick doesn't look much older; he has gained some weight, but he has always been too thin. Doug has aged so much that Ray J. barely recognizes him. He had expected him to meet him with a wisecrack about their last few days together in San Diego, but he actually has tears running down his cheeks as he hugs him.

The years of war created a shortage of goods, and money is scarce. Marilee saved most of the allotment that she received during his tour of duty. His Dad had put aside most of the money he had sent home, so they buy furniture and a used car.

Housing is the biggest problem. All the servicemen are coming home and moving out just as they are. His folks had bought a house and moved back into town some years ago, so they stay with them until they finally find a small house with a living room, bedroom, kitchen, and bath. All the rooms are so small they are almost afraid to sneeze for fear one of them will be blown out of the room. They put Anne's baby bed in the living room so they can have some privacy.

Ray J. finds a job as a trainee with J.C. Penney Company and looks forward to becoming a manager of one of their stores one day. The pay isn't much and the hours are long: eight hours a day for six days and then coming back some nights to learn how to make the signs to put over each table of goods.

Nick and Doug buy a service station on Broad Street, just above the post office. Soon Helen is pregnant, and the two of them rush home to his parents to break the good news. Winnie gets pregnant, but within a month they discover it's in her tubes.

Before they get adjusted to a life of three, Marilee is pregnant with John, their son, and he arrives just ten months after Ray J. returns.

Finding a job, a house, picking out furniture, getting adjusted to civilian life again, especially as a married man with two children, keeps them busy for a few years. It is three years later that Ray J. begins finally to see the woman he had married in such haste.

They are cleaning out a closet of magazines and litter when Marilee loses her temper and smacks him across the face. As an instinct, he hits her with a magazine and then grabs her arms and pulls her down to the floor. He is so shocked by her actions and even more so by his own because their family never experienced abuse in any form.

Marilee says she inherited her moods and her bad temper from her father.

"If you ever hit me again or lay a finger on one of the kids, I will take them and leave you!"

During the next twelve years of their marriage, Ray J. and the kids try to deal with her moods and temper, but she never again strikes any of them.

For a few years they enjoy the good life of working, going to see current movies, and, despite Ray J.'s upbringing, going to dances at the Odd Fellows' Club.

Encouraged by Ray J. and his family, Marilee goes back into training to finish her courses and pass the state exam to become a registered nurse. Going to work as a nurse for a doctor in private practice helps her with her restlessness for a little while. Ray J. takes the civil service exam and begins to work as a postal clerk.

1950's

Having worked for years at Penneys for forty-eight hours a week and more, now Ray J. has an eight-hour shift Mondays through Fridays. Lawrence works full time for his Dad in the furniture business, and they need more help, so Ray J. begins to work on Saturdays.

Poor men, most of them Black, come into the store and ask to speak to Mr. Ray, for they all call their dad "Mr. Ray". They tell him what they need, and his dad looks with them throughout the store until they find whatever it is. He sometimes sells a bedroom suite for $50.00 and lets the guy pay $1.00 down and a $1.00 a week. On top of that, one of them drives out to his house to collect it.

Ray J.'s territory to collect is known as "Rabbit Town". It's across the railroad tracks and everybody who lives there is Black. Marilee tells him that some day a drunken Black man will hit him over the head for the money he is collecting. She just doesn't know that his dad has a reputation among the Black people of their small town and nobody is going to hurt any of them.

Each Saturday morning his dad gives Ray J. the collection cards for the day with instructions on each one:

"Go easy on this one, for they have sickness in the family and it might create a hardship for them to pay their dollar."

Another one,

"Go to the side door and knock and wait until someone hollers for you to give your name. They sell bootleg liquor but don't pay any attention to what is going on."

Sure enough, when he gets to that house with all the cars parked outside, he knocks and gives his name and a deep voice says,

"Let him in. It's ok. It's a Pharr kid."

North Carolina is a "dry" state, which means liquor is controlled by the government and each county decides on whether it will permit liquor to be sold. Iredell County where they live is dry, so people buy bootleg or drive over across the river to Catawa County and buy it. There is a limit on how much one person can buy, so Saturday is a dangerous time to be out on Highway 10 because so many people are going to buy their booze for the week.

To School Again

It becomes evident that their marriage will not work in this small town where both their parents live. Marilee's only sister is a nurse, married, and lives nearby. Ray J. has six siblings, some with their families, living in the same town. Every Sunday is a repeat of the Sunday before: Get up, get dressed, go to church, then on to Marilee's parents for lunch with them and her sister and her family and then back home and to bed. Sometimes he insists that they stop by his parents if only for a short period of time. When they do stop, it always ends the same way,

"I'm ready to go home" very shortly after they get there.

Finally, one Sunday afternoon, Marilee announces she can no longer visit his parents for they make her sick with their hugging and kissing and telling everyone how much they love them and how great they are and on and on. Furthermore, her mother is sick of hearing him talk about his mother being a former schoolteacher. None of her family has even graduated from high school.

"Hell", she says, "Mine only loved my sister, and I got sick of hearing how cute she was, how sweet, how adorable, and what a tomboy I was. The only reason I went into nurse's training was to prove to her that I could do what my sister did."

The following semester Ray J. is a full time student, full time postal worker, married with two children, but determined to find a way to get out of town and make a new life.

They try to keep their troubled marriage from the family but it isn't easy, especially when his sister Emily comes by to visit one afternoon and Marilee answers the door with, "What the hell do you want?" Startled, Emily says she only wants to visit and see the kids.

"I just got the kids to bed for their naps, I'm reading, and I don't want to be disturbed."

With that, she slams the door in her face, and Emily goes home sobbing so hard that her husband Frank thinks someone has died. Even today, so many years after Marilee's death, Emily sometimes reminds Ray J. of that awful afternoon.

◆   ◆   ◆

Lawrence and Mildred with their two children buy a house on North Mulberry Street, just two streets over from Maple Avenue where Ray and Leola moved just before the war broke out. Since they have only one car, Lawrence drives it to work. Lawrence Junior is only two and Velma Jean is a very young baby. Mildred sometimes takes both kids and walks two miles to have a few minutes to talk to Lawrence when he is at work.

Business at the furniture store picks up when materials become available, so Lawrence buys a three-bedroom home on Bost Street. For several years, until Velma Jean gets married, Bost Street is a wonderful place to live. All the neighbors enjoy their privacy, but they are warm and friendly. Judge and Virginia Winberry live just down the street. An attorney and his wife live next to them; two medical doctors live further down the street; the postmaster and his wife live across the street—all decent, hard-working people.

Mildred thrives while living there because all the mothers stay at home with their children, and she is within walking distance of most anywhere in town she wishes to go. Lawrence and Mildred do not socialize much; their lives consist of work, home, and the church. They are completely devoted to one another and their children. With her family being her world, Mildred feels awkward and inadequate outside it. They have great passion in their lives whether it be for loving or for disagreeing with each other. They believe that lives without passion have little substance.

For several years Lawrence Junior and Velma Jean go to school and come home to play in the backyard; Mildred refuses to let them out of her sight.

Graduating from high school, Jean (as she now wants to be called) attends Mitchell College. Lawrence Junior is already attending as a part-time student while he works full time.

At eighteen, Jean has turned into the beauty of the family. Like her grandmother, she has soft skin with rose cheeks, and rich black hair shot through with red highlights. Her lips and tall, fluid build are her grandmother's again. Her eyes are large and shining, drawing the attention of every male she meets. Her breasts are fully developed at an early age, and yet she remains somewhat shy and humble.

Unaware that a young man who has lived down the street from them has been watching her grow up, Jean is surprised when he stops her in front of her house one day with:

"My name is Ray Hartness, and I live in the two-story house on the corner. May I walk you to your door and introduce myself to your mother?"

Impressed with his courtly manners (but more impressed by the fact that he attends Duke University as a medical student), Mildred encourages Jean to date him. They date for a year, and when she completes the semester, they marry. Even though he is five years older than Jean, Mildred is so proud to have a son-in-law to call "Doctor". To the day he dies, she always refers to him as "my son-in-law, the doctor".

After seven years, the marriage ends in divorce. Jean doesn't give a reason or make excuses. He is the father of their three children, and he should have the love of his children as well as the love of her parents.

Death Strikes the Tree

Many people in the Bible belt say that tragedies come in threes. Returning from the beach with his family, Monty is thrown from the car when a drunken soldier hits Doug's van, and he is killed instantly. Doug and Helen are in the hospital for six days with multiple injuries. Within three weeks, Aunt Cal dies in her sleep one night, and Ray dies from an accident.

Lawrence has already left the store and his dad is locking up the back when a man slips up behind and stabs him in the back. With blood flowing freely from the wound, he gets to the phone and calls for help. By the time the ambulance gets him to Long's Hospital, he is dead. All the family rush to see him, but they are too late. Ray J. walks in just as they pull the sheet over his face.

Reverend Grady White, a friend since early childhood, conducts the services at New Hope Baptist Church, and he is buried in Oakwood Cemetery in Statesville.

Grady walks down from the pulpit and talks personally to the children, calling each one by name and assuring them that Ray is in Heaven with his Heavenly Father where he awaits their coming. Turning to Leola,

"Leola, I have known Ray for over fifty years, and you for over thirty. You are the one love of Ray's life. He fell in love with you at first sight and his love continued to grow with each passing year. The church is full, with people standing outside, of relatives and friends who loved Ray—he was that kind of person.

"He will be missed in this life, but the joy of you two meeting in the next life will soon overshadow the short period of time remaining in this one. Your children and grandchildren will continue to surround you with the love that you two instilled in them."

◆   ◆   ◆

Bill and Wanna decide to postpone their wedding plans, but Leola has other ideas. They have already sent out their wedding invitations, the church has been reserved, the cake ordered, dresses have been made, and many wedding gifts have already been received.

"Bill, you know your dad would want you to go ahead with your plans. Life must go on without him. Ask Lawrence, as your oldest brother, to be your best man. You and Wanna go ahead and get married, move in with me, and finish your degree."

Western Avenue Baptist is filled and overflowing before their wedding ceremonies begin. Wanna Sue is radiant in her gown of white flowing behind her as she comes down the aisle on the arm of her father, Fred. Her mother, Beulah, is already in tears before they reach the alter. Her sister, Sherwyn, is almost as beautiful as she.

As Bill stands beside Lawrence, waiting for his bride-to-be to reach them, he has that same wide grin across his face that he had when was only nine years old. They slip away to their undisclosed honeymoon as quickly as their vows are exchanged.

◆   ◆   ◆

Changing his daytime shift to the graveyard, Ray J. enrolls in college again—this time at Lenoir/Rhyne in Hickory—to finish his degree in English to become a schoolteacher. His mother is already looking after Anne and John when they get out of school, so he and Marilee move in with her when Bill and Wanna move to Leesburg, Florida, to teach in an elementary school at Wildwood, Florida, and Wanna has a position with the Citizen's National Bank in Leesburg.

The day finally arrives when Ray J. gets a contract to teach English in a high school in Seminole County, Florida. Marilee wants to sell the house, but he insists that they rent it. His dad had Dad taught them that real estate is always a safe investment. This is the first of many houses that he will buy, as he moves on to other cities to teach, and one day have enough rental houses and apartments to retire.

A nurse can always find a job since there is always a shortage, so Marilee finds a position almost immediately working for a doctor with a private practice. She lets them know that since she works eight hours a day, she will need her rest in the evenings so Anne can cook the meals because all she does is go to school.

1960's

Florida

At the beginning of fall semester, Ray J. enrolls at Stetson University in Deland which is close enough for him to get out of school and meet the classes at 7PM. By taking evening and Saturday classes and going full time in summers, he gets his master's degree in two years.

The moody people of this world should wear a sign that says, in effect,

"I am a moody person, and I woke up this morning in one mood, yours to find out, and I am open to change at any given moment, again yours to find out."

Every morning, Anne and John awake and tiptoe around the house until they find out the mood of their mother. They come home from school and wait for their mother to come home from work. What will her mood be like today? They like it better when their dad is there. He can find out and let them know.

Only too well Anne remembers the times as a teenager when she comes home from school and prepares the evening meal. Will this one please her mother? Not too often would she get a compliment, but quite frequently instead she would hear,

"Too much salt in the beans", or, "Who in the world told you how to cook black-eyed peas, your precious MaMa?"

Having spent months and months working forty hours a week, Ray J. had accepted "headache" and gone to sleep. Now, with somewhat a normal life, he assumes that sex will be normal. Instead, moment of truth:

"I have never enjoyed sex. As a nurse I know it is a biological need. Go ahead and get it over with, but hurry, I need my sleep."

He is thirty-four years old and no one in the family has ever gotten a divorce. If he does, what will happen to the kids? To commit adultery will send him to hell.

Sooooo, life wasn't meant to be a bed of roses. He finds a part-time job working at Belk-Lindsey in the Men's Clothing Department from 4 PM to closing time at 9:30 PM each day after school. He works all day Saturday from 10 AM to 9:30 PM. He gets up early, fixes his breakfast, packs a lunch, gets to school by 8 AM, and teaches until 3:30 PM. After the store closes, each clerk counts his money and turns it in. He usually gets home about 10:30, exhausted, and falls asleep without even thinking about sex.

In all the years they live in Florida, they never have a friend outside of their workplace. Marilee doesn't want friends.

"After I work all day, standing on my feet, I'm too tired to be bothered by anyone. I just want to go to bed with a good book and not be disturbed."

She refuses to go to any of the school functions so Ray J. goes alone to give support to plays, games, and other activities. He grows tired of giving excuses to fellow faculty members for his wife's absences, and they finally quit asking.

Hurricane Hazel

Living in that house for eight years, the only couple to visit them is his brother Bill and his wife, Wanna. When hurricane Hazel is due to come through the area, they come over to stay during the storm.

They cook a ham, a turkey, lots of vegetables, and have plenty of food in the house for they expect the power to be off for days. The day before it is due, they pull the cars into the garage and stuff all lawn chairs and such in around them and close the door. Bill drives his car up tight against the door so the wind won't blow it away.

Winds get up to one hundred fifty miles an hour and they know the eye of the hurricane is near. The power goes off, and they are in darkness except for the candles on the table. They carry mattresses from the bed and spread them out on the living room floor. Now they are all in one room.

"OK, kids, let's pretend we are having a slumber party. Spread a sheet out on the mattress, and let's eat our dinner on the bed."

Opening the windows a little on the east side of the house, they run to the west side to see the "eye" as it goes by.

The power is off for three days. They have more food prepared than they can eat, but at least they live through it without any harm done to them or to the house. Anne and John still talk of the excitement of watching a hurricane and seeing the "eye" up close.

Days creep into weeks, weeks into months, months into years, and so they exist. One weekend Ray J. realizes how horrible life must be for the kids. They come home from school each day to mood swings and sharp words. It is especially hard on Anne because John is the favorite just as Marilee's sister had been in her family.

Shame and remorse almost overcomes him as he thinks of how selfish he has become. He has been thinking only of how to avoid the misery of life with Marilee and overlooking his role as a loving father. On Anne's birthday he buys her a car. When Marilee comes home that day and discovers what he has done, she literally screams,

"You bastard. How could you do that without asking me?"

"It was my money that I made on my part-time job. I don't think Anne should have to wait on the bus at her age."

"Why should she have a car at her age? I never had a car until I married you. If you are going to do stupid things like that, I may as well be living in a motel."

Separation

This is the beginning of the finale to a loveless marriage. They sit down and start planning for their separation. Ray J. moves into the guest bedroom, and Marilee begins to get accustomed to the idea of living alone. They plan to live this way until John graduates from high school. After that, they will live apart because they do not believe in divorce.

Life becomes bearable again in the coming months. Now there are no outbursts of anger, no tension; and, for the first time, they sit quietly on the couch and are honest with one another.

"I must admit that I probably never loved you. It was the times; it was glands thinking instead of brains. Who knows why? We certainly hadn't known each other very long and we have so little in common."

She tells him how much she resents his getting an education for it makes her feel she is beneath him. She admits that she, too, has never loved him. She had married him to get ahead of her sister in having the first grandchild. She just has to lash out with,

"You and your master's degree", "You think you are so damn smart, but how dumb can you be?" "Kids are with you for only a short time, and they go their own way."

How different can two people be in their outlook on family? Ray J. knows that if he loves them and shows it, they will be his forever.

During this period, Marilee and Ray J. spend more time in talking and listening than they have done in all their years of marriage. She tells him of growing up on the county farm. Her parents were poor and hard working. It took years for her dad to become the superintendent of the county home.

Most of her memories are of having a dad with a temper shouting at her mother and of her mother bragging about her sister and always finding fault with anything and everything that Marilee did. She grows up thinking no one loves her, and she can do nothing right. When she married Ray J., she thought by having the first grandchild her parents would finally give her some credit. Her dad did soften through the years, and he learns to control his temper somewhat, but her mother still favors her sister, and will until the day she dies.

A few years earlier they had bought a food and freezer package service from a guy named Bill. Now Bill is somewhat the typical salesman, but he is likeable, recently divorced, and a lonely guy. They invite him to eat with them occasionally. He soon makes himself at home. Quite often Ray J. comes home from his second job, and more and more Bill and Marilee are sitting at the kitchen table playing cards. The kids are in the living room studying.

One weekend Marilee and Ray J. are discussing their living arrangements, and she asks if he thinks it would look ok if she went out on a date with Bill. Ray J. tells her that it's ok with him, and what did she care what anybody else said.

◆   ◆   ◆

Driving through Casselberry, Winter Park, Altamonte Springs, and all the way to Maitland, Ray J. is about to give up on finding a house he can afford when the secretary of Lyman School calls him.

"Ray J., I hear you are looking for a house to buy. If you want an old house that needs some repair, there is one in my neighborhood in Long-wood."

When he sees this house, it reminds him of the house on Maple Avenue: two story, large rooms with high ceilings, and plenty of old-fashioned windows that can be pushed up and down as little or as much as he wants. It needs some repair, but he can afford the down payment on it and do most of the work himself.

The next weekend, he moves his few belongings into it. He can't sleep the first night for it gives him such a strange sensation to be all alone. It dawns on him during the night that he has actually never been alone in his whole life. He grew up sleeping in the same room with either Doug or Nick. He goes from there to the Navy where there are always several people in the room where he sleeps. Tiny and he share a room while he is in training in the Navy. All through the years in service after that he is with somebody every hour of every day. He comes home to a ready-made family, and now he is all alone.

He just cannot sleep! First, he starts thinking about how many nights he has fallen exhausted in bed beside Marilee and wished he were alone.

He gets up and takes another shower, thinking this will relax him, and he can go to sleep. Instead, as he towels down, he begins to get excited with the thought, "I am naked and no one around to see or hear me." For the first time in a long, long time, he pleasures himself until he is exhausted, then falls into a deep, deep sleep.

After school on Monday, he buys the paint and every evening he paints until it grows too dark to see. When he has finished painting everything but the living room, he goes into Orlando and searches the stores until he finds the wallpaper that has the look that he wants. Tall ceilings look good with old-fashioned wallpaper with sort of a faded look about them.

January is the mildest it's been in years, very little wind and sunshine almost every day. Ray J. starts work on the outside of the house and yard. It feels good to be out of the city where he can have trees and grass to mow and bushes to trim.

One weekend he drives to New Symyrna Beach. Nothing like driving on the beach, spreading his towel on the sand, and stretching out to relax with nothing to worry about for a change. He watches the children playing in the sand, building their castles and getting excited about their creation.

When he awakes from his nap, the children have gone home. He watches the tide come in and wash away their works of art. Now the sand is smooth again, no sign of having been disturbed, somewhat like his painting of a wall to cover all the marks that were made by people long ago.

"Wouldn't it be wonderful to have all our mistakes washed away or covered over and leave us pure again as a child", he muses as he watches the grains of sand being pulled back into the sea, now washed clean and ready to start anew wherever the tide takes them.

By Spring Break, Ray J. has finished the painting and repairing of his home, but he has no money to go anywhere for a week. He goes over to the beach again and drives down to a quiet spot where the sand is soft, and he can hear and watch the water. The sounds and smells lure him to sleep, and it's late when he awakens. The tide is coming in with the sounds getting louder and the waves getting higher and higher. He likens them to the harder, rougher times of life, and the soft soothing sounds of the tide going back out as the softer, peaceful moments. The tide comes rushing back in and pushes the sand about, moving it back and then bringing it forward.

"Man is like a grain of sand," he muses, "being pushed about by life upon the land. As he moves from place to place, he becomes, like sand, a part of all that he encounters. He pauses with first one group and then another, picks up from each, and as he moves on he takes a part of each group that he has known with him".

Ray J. and Marilee had agreed that John would live with his mother until he graduates from high school and goes away to college. Poor John. Before the school year ends, he brings his clothes and his books to his dad's house and announces that he is moving in with him; he can no longer live with his mother. Her moods and temper are more than he can tolerate. With Anne away at college, he has no one to talk to, and she has always been there for him.

With less than two years difference in their ages, these two have been more like twins. Their parents learned when they were very young that when they wanted both of them to know something, they only had to tell one. They tell each other everything. That still holds true to this day.

North Carolina

Vivian Lane, a very beautiful young lady of eighteen, with curly hair and blue eyes, is the daughter of the man who ran away with the young high school girl, leaving Vivian and her three sisters with their mother. As a freshman at Mitchell College, she meets Lawrence Junior, who is the grandson of Ray, who bought the furniture that her dad once owned. When she takes him home to meet her mother, they are both met with a cold reception. Mrs. Lane has hated all men since her husband left.

Just the opposite is true when Lawrence Junior takes Vivian home to meet his parents. Lawrence and Mildred love her from the beginning, and Mildred assures her that she is more than welcome to visit at any time.

Despite her mother's pleas, Vivian and Lawrence Junior get married before the school year ends. Vivian continues her education to become a schoolteacher, and Lawrence Junior takes a full-time job to support them.

Lawrence and Mildred have always wanted to move back to the country, and they like Ray J.'s house. Since he rents it, they trade houses. Miss Frances Nicholson, the realtor that Emily works for, takes over the renting of the house on Bost Street.

◆   ◆   ◆

Recovering from the death of Monty, as well as the wounds they receive from the wreck, Doug and Helen with Suzanne, move back into town with Mrs. Gomerry and her family. Doug sleeps in the guest bedroom downstairs, and Helen sleeps with Suzanne in her old bedroom upstairs. The long hours at work and the loneliness of being alone too much causes Doug to start taking drugs to sleep at night. Little by little, the family learns that Doug got hooked on drugs while in the service after he had been shot in the leg. He had managed to stay clean until Monty's death and the troubles that came after that. Helen blames him for the accident.

"You should have seen that drunk coming and somehow gotten out of the way. You caused the death of my son, but I will see to it that you no longer have a daughter. When she is old enough, I will tell her that you were at fault, and she can forget that you ever lived."

Doug never lets himself be angry; he never asks for anything; he never complains, he never scolds. He understands her grief. She does not realize how her words make his heart sink, nor what an effort is needed for him to continue to listen to her.

Finally, the drugs take hold and he tells her: "I can't go on like this. If I leave the house, I won't be back. You won't ever see me again."

"You seem to think that is an awful thing for me. All I can say is good riddance to bad rubbish."

"Then goodbye."

The pain he suffers is no longer anguish, but a sort of soreness, like one might feel after being thrown from a horse, bruised and shaken. Sometimes in the street he sees a woman who looks like Helen so he hurries on to catch up to her, only to find she is a stranger.

Nick drives him to the Veteran's Hospital in Salisbury and commits him. For several months, Nick and Lib Niblock, the office manager at Blackwelder's Furniture Store where Doug has been working, visit him. Doug and Lib have been friends since fourth grade. Doug quit playing the games that children play together and started playing baseball with the boys. Lib teases him that he left her for a boy. He playfully reminds her that at that age she was tall and thin, with narrow hips and the chest of a boy.

Now she has small regular features, blue eyes, and a broad low brow, a type of Greek beauty. One look at her chest and there is no question about her being a boy. Her husband Quinton came home from World War II disabled and has been in and out of hospitals ever since.

When they release Doug from the hospital, Nick finds him a small apartment near downtown, and Lib helps him get it furnished. Winnie gets impatient with him when he calls the house day and night wanting Nick to come over to see him. Charging desertion, Helen files for a divorce and the judge grants it.

Florida

Fred Fisher, the minister of the First Baptist Church which Ray J. and Marilee have attended since moving to Florida, had been an English teacher before becoming a minister. He and Ray J. had bonded from the beginning of their friendship. It has been so easy for Ray J. to be fond of Fred. Every time he makes a slight error in grammar from the pulpit, he immediately looks out through the audience at Ray J. Of course, Ray J. comments as they shake hands at the door,

"Looks like a church of this size could afford a minister who knows how to speak the language."

Ray J. confides in him about his marital problems. When it becomes evident that a divorce just has to happen, he tells Ray J,

"So much of life is a matter of choosing the lesser of two evils. Nothing is all white or all black. Go ahead with the divorce. You are living in sin the way you two are living now."

A fellow teacher from school, Bunny, tells Ray J. to make an appointment with her husband, Phil, who is a lawyer. He will help him get a divorce the cheapest and easiest way possible. He makes the appointment right away. Phil says he will be glad to help him for he knows how underpaid teachers are. He explains that the easiest and quickest way is to take complete blame so Marilee won't contest it. So it is a matter of court record that Ray J. no longer has any interest in sex with his wife, he is indifferent to family life, and so on and so on, and the house and furniture belong to his wife.

No one, not even his family, will know how overjoyed Ray J. is to give away all worldly possessions in exchange to have his kids to myself. There is no way to go back in time, but he makes a vow to himself: "I will devote my life to seeing my kids have the kind of love surrounding them that I enjoyed in the family I grew up with."

Finally, one day Phil calls and says Ray J. is a free man. Almost twenty years are lifted from his shoulders. For the first time, he can go back home to North Carolina and feel comfortable around his family.

So Ray J. breaks the mold: He gets the first divorce in his family. Several others soon follow suit.

The first place Ray J. goes when he gets into town is to see Doug, who is at work. They go up to the second floor where the bedroom suites are on display and crawl up on a bed—the way they used to do as kids. Now, for the first time, Ray J. can pour out his misery with his marriage. Doug lets him get a word or two said when he interrupts with,

"Ray J., you don't have to explain anything to anybody in this family. While you were overseas and Marilee was living with her parents, Mother and Dad used to drive down to see her and Anne. They reported to the rest of the family how they were doing. After only a few visits, Dad said to me, 'Doug, be sure you stay close to your brother in the years to come for he is going to have a rough life with that woman'."

With such relief, Ray J. begins to cry in his brother's arms. He knew that his family would always support him, but, still, getting a divorce was considered to be a sin. To be held once again by a loving member of his family brings wracking sobs. He remembers his dad's arms around him, holding him so tight, when he left home for the first time, and every time he came home and left.

Not everything is perfect, even in his own family. On his next trip to North Carolina it's his turn to spend the night with Lawrence and Mildred. When he awakes the next morning, both of them have gone to work. He wanders out to the kitchen to get a bowl of cereal. As he sits down at the kitchen table to eat, he finds a Bible opened with a note that says,

"Ray J., please read the passage from the Bible that tells us it is a sin for a man to divorce his wife. Remember, if you should ever want to marry again, you and your wife will be living in sin all of the days of your lives."

It is signed: "Your loving sister-in-law who loves you and wants to meet you in heaven some day."

Irony, poetic justice, whatever, in just a few years first her daughter then her son will divorce their spouses and marry again. Some years after that, her son will divorce and marry the third time. In the final marriage of each, they find their soul mates at last.

Just three weeks after her divorce, Marilee and Bill get married by a justice of the peace. Marilee quits her job as a nurse, and she and Bill open a small appliance shop over in Coco Beach. Maybe now Marilee will be happy with a man who is with her twenty-four hours a day and can give her his complete attention.

Sadly, this marriage ends in a divorce in less than a year. Marilee finds a job with another doctor in a private practice. By this time, Ray J. has moved to California but Marilee never discussed her breakup with Bill nor his sudden death within a few months. Much later, he learns from Anne that Bill was an alcoholic, he was diabetic, and he had physically abused her.

New Growth on Limbs

North Carolina

Bob is now a young man of twenty-two with brown hair through which he passes his hand frequently with a careless gesture. His eyes are brown, very large, and they look tired most of the time. He is clean-shaven at all times, and his mouth, not withstanding thin lips, is well shaped. People notice how perfect his skull is—the head of a thinker. He is tall and thin and holds himself with a deliberate grace. Leola often looks at him when he is starring intently at his books and thinks how much he makes her think of pictures of her dad when he was that age.

Bob is a good listener; though he often thinks of clever things to say, it is seldom that he says them. Sometimes he surprises everyone when he makes a subtle crack about someone or something. Most of the time he sits quietly, lost in thought, but his greatest quality is a vitality which seems to give health to everyone whom he comes in contact with. He loves people of all ages, occupations and purposes and often listens to the failures as well as the successes of their lives.

One day while looking at Jean and Ray's wedding pictures, he stares intently at one of the bridesmaids.

"Jean, who is the beautiful girl with the clean, fresh look standing next to you?"

"That is one of my best friends, Judy Webb. Uncle Bob, you want me to fix up with a date with her?" she teases.

Several days later, he finds that Judy has transferred to Women's College in Greensboro, but she comes home quite often to be with her parents, John Henry and Edith. After several attempts, she finally agrees to go out with him to a movie.

For years, Judy had planned to enroll in Women's College, but in her initial physical examination, the doctors discovered that she is diabetic. John Henry and Edith insist that she attend Mitchell College and commute from home while they check the adjustment to the medication. Otherwise, she would not have attended Michell and been in Jean's wedding.

The weeks pass into months, Bob takes a position at the high school in Troutmans, teaching science courses and coaching baseball while Judy finishes her degree in home economics.

Trying out for the Houston Colts, Bob is given a one-year contract. When the year is up, they offer him a long-term contract, but he doesn't want to be away from Judy. He returns home.

With Judy spending the summer at home with her parents, life is wonderful! They see each other every evening and sometimes during the day. One evening she is cooking the meal while her parents are shopping. Bob is very nervous; he does not know where to begin. At last, he cannot bear it any longer.

"Judy, would you join hands with me and start on life's journey together? You and I can have a wonderful, joyous journey together until some day we reach our final destination."

The following day there are no clouds in the sky, and the air is sweet and clean. They are at the tennis courts. Bob observes how well she wears her clothes, so elegant beside the others.

"Green suits you," she says. "You look nice today." He blushes with delight and hardly knows what to say.

"Thank you. I can honestly return the compliment. You look perfectly beautiful." She smiles and gives him a long look with her green eyes.

Bob is very fond of tennis. He serves well, plays close to the net, and it is difficult to get a ball past him. He very easily wins all his sets. They make it a practice of walking together every afternoon, so when the last set is over, Bob insists they go for a walk.

"Haven't you had enough exercise for one day?" she asks. "The stars are all out," he says.

He is in high spirits. He puts his arms around her and kisses her lips. She only laughs a little but doesn't pull away.

"You must not do that," she says. "And why not?" "I like it," she laughs.

From this point on, things are entirely different between them. She says things no woman has said to him. She compliments him. She says his eyes fascinate her. His lips are sensual; and when he kisses her, it is wonderful to experience a passion she has never known she is capable of feeling. He kisses her a great deal. It is so much easier to do that than to find the words to express his love for her. Sometimes he flings his arms around her without warning; and, caught off guard, she laughs and blushes, but surrenders herself willingly to his passion.

Lying in bed, he cannot sleep for thinking about her. He has always thought that love was full of rapture—an ecstatic happiness that brings peace. Instead, he now has a painful yearning, almost anguish, to be beside her every moment of his life. His last thoughts before going to sleep are of taking her in his arms, kissing her full red lips, and running his fingers down her spine.

When he tells his mother that he wants to marry Judy, Leola gives him some advice:

"Bob, Judy may some day have some health problems due to her diabetes. Make sure you love her because she will depend on you entirely at that time in your lives. Do you realize that you two should never have children; it's too dangerous?"

"I love Judy far more than I could possibly love a child of mine. We have already discussed it. Judy is concerned that I may want children, but I have convinced her that I don't."

Knowing how protective Edith and John Henry are about their daughter, he is prepared to answer their questions when he tells them of his desire to marry Judy.

"Mother has already told me of the dangers that may be in store for Judy. I promise you that I will take care of her if bad times do come along. She and I joined hands, hearts, and lives some time ago. If the sea that we sail becomes rough, we will continue to sail together until we reach the other side."

New Salem Methodist Church has been home for Judy since she was a young child. She and Bob talk with her minister about marriage, their commitment to one another, and the arrangements for their wedding. June 4th is the date they agree upon.

When Bob calls Ray J. and asks him to take part in his wedding to Judy, Ray J. is overjoyed. He immediately makes plans to drive to North Carolina. Fortunately, the wedding is scheduled for June, and school will be out for the summer.

Arriving in Statesville, he is embarrassed to tell Bob that he doesn't have a suit of clothes suitable to wear in the wedding. Luckily, he and Bob are about the same size, so Bob gives him a light blue suit that he can wear as well as take home for Bob has several others. The irony that Ray J. sometimes resented having to wear "hand-me-downs" from his older brothers while a teenager and now as an adult very grateful to be wearing a "hand-me-up" from a younger brother.

John Henry walks down the aisle escorting Judy in her white dress with her niece as the flower girl. Bob stands waiting with his brother Bill as his best man, his best friend, Bill Hugglie, and his brother Ray J. beside him.

In the motel, Judy tells him: "Wait for me. I will be out of the bathroom in a little while."

Bob's heart is beating wildly, a strange feeling of happiness he has never felt before. He is convinced of her purity, of her heart so full of charity. Her lips are soft and full against his. He closes her eyes with kisses on her eyelids, first one, then the other. A lump suddenly fills his throat and tears come into his eyes.

Florida

Taking his mother back home with him, Ray J. is delighted to turn the running of the house over to her. He doesn't remember when he could eat his breakfast and walk out the house and go to school with someone to wash the dishes, make the beds, and clean the house.

"You have no idea how great it feels to be able to take over the kitchen after all these years", Leola tells him. "That is one of the things I miss the most about living in someone else's house."

After four months of observing how much his mother misses being among her relatives and friends, Ray J. takes her back to Statesville. They search the newspapers and find a small apartment just three blocks down East Broad Street within walking distance of a grocery store. Ray J. sleeps on the couch for the next three nights and then returns home.

California

"Life begins at forty" may be true for some people, but for Ray J., it begins at forty-one. He finishes the school year and draws out his retirement. He and the two kids pack their clothes in two cars and head for California. They aren't the "Joads" from Steinbeck's Grapes of Wrath who took so long to get to California, but they have all they own in two cars.

Eight days of singing and exploring this country that his kids have never seen makes him feel like a kid again. All his life he has loved it with all its faults and mistakes. He still stands stiff with pride whenever he sees the flag or hears the National Anthem.

Interstate 10 is just being built so they have many side trips along the way. They didn't know how much warmer the water is along the white sand of Sarasota. They marvel at just how majestic the old houses of Gulfport, Mississippi, appear on the right side of the highway with the water on the left. One day they hope to come back and explore New Orleans, but this trip they don't have the time or money.

Just before they reach Texas, the heavens open and they have a downpour like none they have seen before. They slow down to ten miles an hour when the hail starts peppering the windshields. They can barely see the car in front of them.

Creeping into Beaumont, Texas, they're greatly relieved to find a cheap motel. Ray J. has to admit the kids are right when they complain about all that "nothing" they see between Beaumont and El Paso. Years later when they live in Waco, they discover that most Texans won't admit that El Paso is really Texas; they swear it belongs to Mexico.

Las Cruces, New Mexico, is a sight for sore eyes. All the beauty of a sleepy town so spread out that it is hard to believe how many people live there. Ray J. wonders if Las Cruces is the only "Land of Enchantment". The stretch between it and Tucson, Arizona, has nothing but heat, snakes, and bugs. When the windshield is almost covered with the bugs that have hit it, John says,

"At least there are about 50 bugs that won't have the guts to hit anybody else."

They spend their last night on the road in Phoenix, Arizona, where the temperature is 115 degrees that day. Getting up early, they hurry to get out of that heat before the sun gets up too high.

Arriving in Santa Ana, California, without a job and money running low doesn't bother Ray J. all that much. He had walked away from tenure in Florida. The few friends he had made told him how foolish it was to turn his back on security like that, but he thinks,

"Thank God my parents gave me the roots to feel secure within myself and faith that I can take whatever the next day brings. All the times I have heard, 'And wings to soar like an eagle' rings in my ears."

Within a few days Ray J. is working at Disneyland as a security guard at night, and John gets a job at one of the food stands as a bus boy. Anne goes back to continue her education at the University of South Florida in Tampa.

John enrolls at Santa Ana Community College for $15 for his parking sticker plus books. His bosses at Disneyland work out a schedule for him each semester. He continues to work there until he graduates from Chapman College over in Orange.

Just as Ray J. is beginning to think that he will be working at Disneyland for the year, and three days after school starts, he get a call from the Placentia District. He signs a contract to teach remedial reading at Kraemer Immediate School in the mornings and development reading at Valencia High School in the afternoons. Luckily they are back to back so he can walk from one to the other in about ten minutes.

Three thousand miles away from anyone they know, John and his dad grow in their love for one another and form a friendship unsurpassed by any other outside their marriages later on. They pool their money to pay expenses and to send money to Anne so she can continue her education.

Joan

Life continues to be good to Ray J. as he signs a contract for a full-time English teacher at the high school for the next year. What a large school with over one hundred teachers with fifteen in the English department alone!

In addition to his teaching assignment, Ray J. is assigned to be the advisor to the Yearbook. Emily Bisen is the advisor to the school newspaper, so the two of them are often at school in the evenings with the students who work on the two publications.

Within a month after school starts that year, Ray J. begins to feel that he belongs when he is invited to join the bowling league. They bowl every Friday after school. In years to come, he jokingly tells everyone,

"I gave up bowling, for here was the place I met Joan."

The two of them are placed on the same team so it becomes a habit for them to finish bowling and stop at the bar. Each time, Ray J orders a screwdriver and nurses it for a long time and eventually gets it down. After a few weeks, they often eat at the restaurant in the bowling alley if John is not going to be home that evening.

Most people at school assume that Ray J. is married because he still wears his wedding band and talks about his two kids. He begins to tell Joan about his past. She is twenty-five and has never been married, but her family is beginning to drop gentle hints. She received her degree in business, economics and political science at UC, Boulder, and moved to Garden Grove to teach. After two years, she moved back home and got her master's degree in counseling at UNC at Greeley. She returned to California and taught business courses at La Habra High last year. By coincidence, she gets the position of counselor the same year Ray J. arrives on the scene. So many ships pass in the night but theirs were meant to be in the light of day. Ray J. is eighteen years older than she so he looks upon her as a kid sister.

Eating in a restaurant is an expense Ray J. can't afford too often. He tells Joan they will have to skip that part of their Fridays. She is a very persuasive person and convinces him to let her buy her own meals and he buy his. He is not comfortable with doing that because gentlemen don't do that back home. But since he has to eat somewhere and she says she hates to eat alone, he agrees to it.

One Saturday they drive over to Redondo Beach to see her grandmother, Muncher. On the way over she tells him that "Muncher" is the name everyone calls her and her other grandmother is called "Murmur". Two old ladies in their eighties couldn't be more different, according to Joan. Murmur is "Crab Apple Annie", and Muncher is the sweetest thing this side of heaven. She and "Pa" have lived in Mesa, Arizona, for most of their lives, but Muncher cannot stand the heat. For the past thirty some years she spends October through April in their home in Mesa and April to October in a little rented house on Redondo Beach.

They arrive right at lunchtime and Muncher has her friend, Loretta, and a young couple to lunch. Soon after they finish eating, everyone leaves, so they have time for Muncher and Ray J. to get acquainted. It is "love at first sight" for he is overwhelmed by her charm and her acceptance of modern day life. She announces that the young couple is not married, just living together, but it is ok for people live that way over here on the beach.

The next time they visit her, she is excited about a movie that she and Loretta have seen. They usually take a bus to do their shopping and go to movies and such for neither one can drive. This one particular day there is no bus available when they want to get to the movie so Muncher steps out on the street and thumbs a ride. Some old gentleman picks them up and drives them directly to the movie. She cautions,

"Don't you dare tell Corinne. She would have a fit to know I hitchhike a ride when I'm over here. What she doesn't know won't hurt her. The movie had Warren Beatty and Julie Christie in it, and Loretta and I nearly died laughing at the things they say in movies nowadays. I didn't know you could talk about being a whore in movies, but they certainly did in this one."

Sometime later when Ray J. meets Joan's mother and dad, he finds it hard to believe that Muncher is the mother of Corinne. One so open to ideas and people of all races and the other so closed minded and sheltered from the realities of life by her husband.

During the coming months, Joan and Ray J. begin to see each other on weekends and attend movies and ball games together. One weekend they go to Las Vegas and play the slots and attend some of the shows.

The night they see Englebert Humperdink in a nightclub in Las Vegas sitting in a chair on stage begin to sing *Amazing Grace*, they sit spellbound. As he continues to sing each verse, he slowly starts rising. When he stands tall and his voice reaches its peak, the audience gives the most thunderous applause they have ever heard in any place in their lives. When the show is over, they walk out feeling as if they have been in a church.

They include one of the teachers from school who is single on one of their trips, and soon he becomes a third every time they go to Vegas. John DeMike is the speech teacher from school and a most unusual person. He was born without arms and legs but had a normal size body. He said his parents took him home after the hospital admitted they didn't know what to do with him and his mother told his dad, "Let's feed it and see what happens."

Now he is twenty-nine years old and has had so many operations he quit counting. A wonderful sense of humor like no other, John tells everyone at school that Ray J. and Joan take him with them because they know they take them up front at the shows, and they don't have to wait in line. At the first faculty meeting, Dave, the principal, asks each person to stand when called and tell something about his life. When he calls upon John, he replies,

"You want me to sit here where everyone can see me, or try to stand and disappear below the table?"

For the remainder of their years in California, John remains one of their best friends (one of the few invited to their wedding). They love him like a brother.

At school one day, Emily asks everybody for reactions about an occasional meeting with the Language Department, for the chairs of Spanish and French have asked her to consider it. Usually, Ray J. hates meetings, but he is glad they decide to meet for here he meets Susan, one of the few friends that Joan and Ray J. makes that continues to be in their lives after almost fifty years. Susan is a damn Yankee from New Jersey, as Ray J. still reminds her, (and she still teaches Spanish and ESL at a college in Oregon). She is dating a guy by the name of Wayne who teaches Russian at La Habra High School. When Ray J. tells her that he is seeing Joan, the new counselor, and she used to teach at La Habra, the four of them meet for dinner one evening. This dinner marks the beginning of a friendship that has lasted through the years.

By the time spring arrives that first year, Joan and Ray J. are known as a couple and are invited to join in several community activities. One evening while attending a concert with another couple, Nellie and Burch, they run to the car in the rain and jump into the back seat. Joan is cold and snuggles up to get warm so Ray J. puts an arm around her. As she begins to get warm, he begins to get hot and realizes that he is no longer having brotherly feelings about her. She is feeling the same way. They are both surprised at this turn of events. When they get to her apartment, they sit on the couch and talk most of the night.

The next day at school, he can hardly wait to tell Ken, a friend and only other male in the English Department. He thinks it will be a big surprise but, instead, Ken laughs and says he and his wife, Sue, have been waiting to see how long it would take him and Joan to realize the obvious.

It seems there are several teachers across campus who have seen them together several times and have wondered the same thing. Later, they find out the secretaries of several departments have a pool going about when Joan will get pregnant.

One night there must have been a full moon and the stars were shining brightly and the heavens collided when Ray J. has sex with a woman who enjoys it and actually participates in the rhythm and joy of two bodies becoming one. The next day Ray J. returns home, packs his clothes, and moves in.

The next few months are the happiest of his life. Working in the same school, rushing home to each other to discover how perfectly matched they are in every way; even the difference in their ages disappear.

Anne marries Arnold, the guy she has been dating since high school. Suddenly, John decides he can't wait until he graduates so he and Paula get married. Under the GI bill, Ray J. buys a four-bedroom house with pool on a large lot in Anaheim, so John and Paula move in with Joan and his dad. Everything should have been prefect; except, Ray J. has a tinge of guilt about living with someone without marriage.

Earthquake

Early one morning before they get out of bed, the house begins to shake. Pictures come off the walls and fall to the floor. The sound of breaking glass is heard in every room. It lasts for only a few seconds but the mess it leaves takes hours to clean up later in the day. They turn on the radio and learn the earthquake that hit them did minor damage compared to what it did in Long Beach.

Anne in Florida

Ray J. can hardly wait for summer to arrive so he can get back to Florida to see Anne and Arnold. He had not been able to come to Anne's graduation from college nor their wedding, but Marilee is there with them for both. No one, even Marilee, believes that Anne's Grandmother Sherrill sends her a lone dollar bill for her graduation from college. She is the first person in the entire Sherrill family to get a college degree.

Marilee had met Jim, who is the city manager of the town and, according to Anne, it is a stormy marriage from the beginning.

After driving for three long days, and it's very late, Ray J. arrives in town and finds their small apartment. Anne is ironing the outfit that she will be wearing for the activities of the next day. She is working in the summer program. She stops immediately when he rings the doorbell and greets him with tears in her eyes, but how great it is to hug her and kiss away the tears.

She tells him to sit on the couch so they can talk while she finishes ironing. He asks why she can't wear something else the next day and let the ironing wait. In a faltering voice she says she has only one outfit so she has to wash it out each evening, dry it, iron it, and wear it again the next day. He jumps from the couch,

"Why in the world do you have only one outfit? You have taught all winter and now you work in the summer program, and no money?"

Then she tells him the arrangements that she and Arnold have worked out. While she teaches junior high English and grades papers and prepares for the next day, Arnold is in graduate school and has more time so he took over their finances. He put her on a budget and so she just doesn't have the extra money for clothes. Ray J. pretends to understand, and they spend the remainder of the evening getting her clothes ready for the next day. He first tells her about his life with John and Paula. Then he tells her about Joan, since they have never met.

It grows late, and he is tired so he asks her,

"When will Arnold be home?"

"He often stays out late with friends for they need to study. Arnold says graduate level courses are just harder and require a lot more study than undergraduate."

They make out the couch, and he soon falls asleep and doesn't know when or if Arnold comes home. He hears noises in the morning but doesn't get off the couch because he had been uneasy during the night and had not slept well at all. Anne finally taps him on the shoulder and says,

"Sorry, Dad, but I have to leave for work. I'll try to be home early so we can talk."

Half awake, he tells her that he is on a time frame and has to leave for North Carolina that day but has scheduled two days with her on his way back. They hug, she cries as usual, and then leaves. Ray J. quickly goes to the bathroom and gets dressed for it is over seven hundred miles to North Carolina.

Ray J. has had better visits with his family in North Carolina: his mind keeps coming back to Anne's situation. There are just too many things about her working, his handling the money, her having only one outfit, his staying out late with friends, that crock about graduate courses being so hard (been there, done that).

He is anxious to get back and see them face-to-face and find out more about their marriage. He plans to arrive Friday afternoon, have the weekend when she isn't working, and then leave early Monday morning for home.

When he arrives, Anne is home but Arnold isn't. Furthermore, he doesn't come home by midnight so Ray J. almost demands to know some answers. Sobbing, Anne confesses,

"Oh, Dad. I have been so miserable for most of the past year. I have known Arnold since high school and thought I knew him quite well. Last fall I started teaching and he got into graduate school, but then he turned into a stranger. He got in with guys who studied together at night and they started smoking pot. He soon took over the money and began to tell me how much smarter guys were for they went on to graduate school and the girls became school teachers."

He doesn't come home that night. It is a good thing he didn't. Ray J. might have killed him he was so angry. The next morning they pack her clothes, and he takes her back to California with him.

They have three days in the car to talk, and Anne needs someone to talk with. It is not easy to build up people's confidence in themselves when someone else has had a year to break it down. It certainly helps when they arrive home. John grabs his sister and they hug and kiss and cry until Ray J. has to remind them there are others present.

A Wedding

From the very beginning, there is no jealousy between or among the two kids and Joan. Anne is only five years younger and John a little over six. Their relationship has not been one of mother and kids nor one of siblings, but one so special there are no comparisons to give it. Joan moved into their lives with such love and ease, how could anyone ever resent her? As a matter of fact, it is Anne who comes to Ray J. one day, sits down beside him and asks,

"Dad, when are you and Joan going to get married?"

Caught off guard, he stammers a bit as he inquires about her feelings as well as John's (He knew Anne would know how he felt).

"I think Joan loves you too much to continue living this way, and you should get married. You know John and I love her to death and so do you."

They plan a church wedding with all of Joan's family there. John is to be the best man and Anne the maid of honor. They get married on March 29th, Anne's birthday is the 31st, and Paula gives birth to Lisa May 4th. On Spring Break they take a brief honeymoon at Carmel. They are in the sauna when the door flies open and in walk Wayne and Susan laughing so hard Susan is crying. They knew where they were to stay, so they had followed on their honeymoon. Now, after almost half a century, those four are still best friends and no matter how much time in between their meeting, within five minutes it's as if they have never been apart.

North Carolina

Doug goes back to work with Blackwelder's Furniture Store. Thelma, Norris's wife, insists that Norris take him back in his former position of manager of the store. She has become dependent upon Doug for his advice in handling Dorothy, their young daughter. Norris has spoiled her rotten by giving her everything she asks for; now she is sometimes rude to her own mother.

Arranging her schedule so they have the same lunch hour, Lib goes to lunch with Doug to see that he eats the right foods and stays healthy. She also wants to see that he doesn't get back into taking drugs.

At lunch one day, she reaches over to get a piece of bread at the same time he does. Their hands touch; he looks across the table at her as he takes her hand is his.

"Lib, I have the strangest feeling as I hold your hand. Will you ever think of me as anything but a friend?"

"Doug, I have known you forever it seems. No. You are my best friend. I gave up thinking of anyone other than Quint when I married him. Now, he is more like a brother than a husband. He needs me. Whenever he gets tired of being in the hospital, he knows he can always come home me and our son, Lynn."

"I worry about you. You have a husband to look after when he comes home, and a mother who needs you even if she is in a nursing home. From now on, I will go with you to lift her when you give her the sponge baths. That is the least I can do. Every day doing that will soon give you backaches."

After three years of lifting Mrs. Scott from her bed to her chair and then back to bed, Doug has the backaches. The staff does a good job of keeping her room clean and doing whatever they can to help her, but Mrs. Scott often won't eat until Lib gets there to feed her.

One day at work, Lib comes to Doug, and with a scarlet face, asks if he will speak with her after work. He goes to her at the closing of the store.

"Will you walk with me?" she says, looking away with embarrassment.

They walk around the store and down into the parking lot with neither one saying a word. They get back to the front of the store and sit in a swing on display before she asks,

"Do you remember what you asked me one day at lunch about three years ago? We were at Redmon's Café and our hands touched when we reached for a biscuit."

"Yes, I remember it well. You notice I never mentioned it again."

"Doug, I wasn't completely honest with you. I didn't lie. I guess it was a sin of omission. I have always been drawn to you."

She puts her hand on his shoulder as she speaks, and he reaches over and takes it to his lips.

"Why did you do that?" she asks, with a blush.

"Do you object?" he asks.

He takes her by the elbows and draws her toward him. When she makes no resistance, he kisses her on the lips. He looks into her eyes and sees them soften and glow. Something stirs in his heart and tears appear in his eyes.

"Lib, are you telling me that you love me?"

He draws her to him again, puts his arms around her, and kisses her again and again as she blushes and surrenders herself to him.

"I am so proud, so happy, and so grateful", he tells her as she settles into his arms, and they gently rock back and forth in the swing. This is the beginning of a happiness that will continue until they both die.

1970's

Hawaii

Later that summer, Ray J. and Joan go to Hawaii where they spend their days in a rented car touring the islands and their nights at the Royal Hawaiian Hotel. Each morning they follow the tour bus until they come to a place or site they want to investigate, and then they leave the tour.

They visit three other islands and find one with a little cove that has a small lake with water so clear they can see their feet as they walk in it. Lying on the small beach, looking at the surroundings, they feel they are the only two people on earth. They still remember this day, this island, and this feeling as their true honeymoon.

Having spent many days and nights on these islands during the war when his outfit came here for their R & R, Ray J. begins to tell Joan some of the horrors of being in a war. He recalls seeing his first dead American soldier lying in the path, and having to drive on to his job of the day without stopping. The most chilling picture he carries is of seeing his best buddy step on a mine. There is nothing left to pick up, not even his dog tag.

"Nature or God or some force steps in to help most veterans after having such experiences. Time dims the horrors and at the same time makes more vivid the lighter, brighter side of those years. How clearly I remember Miss Fennel, the American school teacher who used to invite small groups of us to her home for a meal and an evening of relaxing in a home away from home."

The Placentia School District where they work has a policy of no married couples, so Ray J. applies to the Fullerton District. He gets references from Dr. David Tansey, his principal, and Emily, his chair. With their glowing comments, he goes for the interview and is offered a contract for the coming school year. A few days later, Dave calls him into his office and asks him to tear up that contact and stay with his position. When he asks about the policy, Dave tells him,

"Some policies are outdated and should be ignored. Good teachers are more important than policies."

Before their first anniversary, Ray J. realizes that Joan will never feel complete until she becomes a mother. Knowing she will be a different kind of mother and being a parent will not be his responsibility alone, he is eager to be a father again. What a disappointment when she cannot get pregnant. Worried and fearing the worst, he sees the doctor to be checked. What a relief when nothing is wrong with his sperm count, and he says it is just a matter of time.

Lisa is two years old and naturally she has to have a sibling. It becomes a race between Joan and Paula who will deliver first. Rachael is born October 17th, and Joan had wanted her delivery to be in October since both she and Ray J. are October babies.

Dave, Joan's principal, is a man far ahead of his time. Even though the district policy states that a pregnant woman has to resign her position at the end of the fifth month, Joan remains on the job until she is over eight months. Again, Dave breaks with policy. As he explains,

"Joan, a counselor, of all the personnel in the school, should be the one to let kids see that we are human, we do have babies, and we are not ashamed of it!"

One day he drops by her office and tells her,

"Perhaps you should stay home until the baby is born. Some of the teachers have been teasing me that I might be the doctor to deliver you."

November eight, their daughter Heather is born. Seeing the look on Joan's face as she feeds her breast to their child makes Ray J. realize just how much he loves his wife. Thinking back to the first time he had seen those beautiful breasts, he had reached down and run his hands over them, caressed them, bent down and kissed them. Now, no thought of sex, just so much in love with the mother and so proud to be the father of their child. *How do I love thee, Let me count the ways* will have more and more meaning for him during the coming years as first one breast is removed because of cancer and then later the other.

Knowing how peer pressure in southern California has influenced so many kids, Ray J. and Joan begin their plans to leave the area. Their school has been a "target school" for the Brown Beret movement. They feel it is not safe to bring Heather to school any more. Gates to the parking lots are now being locked during school hours, and guards are hired to patrol the school grounds. In fact, the building where Joan works is bombed the summer after they leave.

For years Ray J. has wanted to get his Ph.D. and teach at the university level. They think at first that Joan should get a position as a counselor, and they can make it that way. Thinking it through, they see how difficult it might be if he gets his degree and takes a position where she can't get hers. They withdraw both their retirements and decide to tighten their belts and both go to school in Colorado near her parents. Everybody tells them how foolish they are to throw away tenure and good salaries; however, life is more than money and job security.

John in Kentucky

With ambition to teach religion in a small college or university, John and Paula move to Lexington, Kentucky. John has been accepted into the seminary. Going to school again and becoming a minister of a small rural church is exciting and rewarding for John. On the surface, he thinks it is the same for Paula. She brings the kids to church and everyone adores them. But, Paula is having more and more days of being depressed and seems to lack the ability to overcome them. One day John calls and asks his dad to come for a visit once summer is here.

Unaware that things are as bad as they are, Ray J. and Joan take their time in going to Kentucky and stop in North Carolina for a brief visit with family once again. When they arrive in Lexington, no one answers the door even though they hear the radio blasting away. Ray J. opens the door and they walk in.

He looks at Joan and she looks at him in disbelief. It looks as if they have stepped into a horror movie scene. Little Rachael is crawling across the floor in a mess that isn't fit for a pig; sopping wet, dirty, and something in her mouth that Joan immediately takes out and throws away. While Joan is undressing her, Ray J. looks through the apartment and finds Paula in bed with the covers over her head. He hears Lisa whimpering, locked in a closet.

By the time John gets in from school, they have the place somewhat presentable but Paula is still not completely with them. They hug and kiss and say the usual but John looks terrible; exhausted and worn down. He tells them that going to school, studying to keep prepared for his classes, visiting the people in his small congregation, preparing and delivering his sermons on Sundays, has left him little time to devote to Paula and the girls. Then he admits that he simply does not know what to do for someone who is depressed.

They spend three days washing dirty diapers that have been thrown into a corner and discarding dozens that are beyond saving. Joan has long talks with Paula and tells her she must make some changes in her life if she wants to save her marriage and family. Paula insists she has no control over the way her life is going and cannot do a thing about it. Joan then tells her something that not even Ray J. knows about her. She, Joan, has suffered from depression for years although not as severe as Paula.

"I usually go into a quiet place and meditate. If that doesn't pull me out, then I go to a counselor who helps me through it."

Colorado

John realizes they cannot continue with these conditions. He makes a dramatic change in their lives by giving up his dream of teaching religion. He decides he will go back with them to Colorado to prepare for teaching special education.

They rent a large truck, and all chip in with loading their possessions into it. Worn and weary, they make their way across country to Colorado and put John's possessions in storage.

Looking for a three-bedroom apartment in a university town is like looking for a needle in a haystack. John is busy getting all the paper work done to enable him to enroll for the fall semester. Joan and Ray J. go through newspapers and ads, and finally through an agency, trying to find a place to live.

In desperation they turn to the buying section, for surely there must be some run-down place they can afford. Someone up there is looking after them for they find a small house just three blocks down from the university. Using their retirement money, they make a down payment and go back to Loveland as excited as a kid with a new toy.

Joan's dad, Virg, a retired grocer from Safeway, has been building "spec" houses to supplement his income (his dad was a builder and he has long desired to build his own house). He cannot believe anyone can buy a house in one short day.

Although it is already dark, he insists that they take him back to see this "bargain" they have found. When they get there and look it at again from the outside in the dark, it truly looks dismal. Virg has brought a lantern so they go inside to look it over. It has a nice sized living room with a bedroom on the right side and a dining room through glass doors going back to the kitchen and bathroom. It even has a tiny breakfast nook.

Going down a half flight of stairs that lead to the outside, the stairs going down the other half flight go into a small hall with a room and bath that was probably meant to be a guest bedroom. Then there are some more rooms with nothing but the floor and scaffold.

"You two must live with the gods. This is going to turn out to be a good deal. It isn't something I would consider for us for I would never put my wife in such a place. But, considering it is temporary and there are so many of you involved, we can make it work. There is room for you, Joan, and Heather on the first floor. Before school starts we can make that basement into a place large enough for John and his group. We can turn the downstairs bedroom into a living room and finish those other rooms into bedrooms and a kitchen."

Virg, Joan's brother Tom, John, and Ray J. take no time at all to do just what Virg said they could. They are in that house two weeks before school begins. What a happy semester they look forward to with Joan and Ray J. in the doctoral program and John in the Master's Program. Paula has started college so many times (dropped out each time) so she says she will look after the kids.

Never count your chickens until the eggs are hatched. Not even six weeks into the semester and John calls his dad and Joan down to their living room. He and Paula are sitting on the couch looking really weird. When asked what is wrong, Paula seems almost pleased with herself when she says,

"I got tired of looking after kids all day while you three were having fun in your classes with so many people. Today, when I bought the groceries, a good-looking kid carried them to the car, and I went home with him and we had sex. And I am not ashamed of it, for he was a lot better in bed than John has been for a long time."

The next few months are unsettling for everyone. John files for a divorce but fears the judge will give the kids to Paula. He has the reputation of siding with the mother every time. Paula's mother, Alma, says she will testify in court, if necessary, for John to get the girls. She knows they will be better off with him.

When the judge awards the girls to John, there is great rejoicing. Even Paula is relieved, for she just wants to run away from all the problems of the past few years. In fact, she doesn't come back into the picture for the next ten years. Joan will always remember how aghast she feels as Paula walks away even as she, Joan, is holding Lisa with a temperature of 103.

The following months are filled with juggling acts as the three of them continue going to school and at the same time looking after three little girls. They immediately get organized and, as Shakespeare says, *Life becomes a stage and each one plays his part,* as Joan takes on the role of mother to all three girls, and Ray J. and John switch from one role to another as the need arises.

John finds a day care center where they can take them if they have an emergency, but, luckily, they have to use it only once that trimester. Their courses are scattered throughout the day as well as the night so someone is at home with the kids every hour. Whoever is home must be the mother or the father so they learn quickly how to change diapers, wipe runny noses, and how to potty train little girls. Any one of them can use a hammer, change a tire, cook a meal, iron a dress, and even sew on a button if needed.

Just when they think they have everything so organized and each one knows what to do and when throughout the day, October arrives. It starts snowing the last week of October, and they don't see the ground until the middle of February. Not that it snows every day, but one snow comes before the other one melts. They shovel enough snow that winter to last a lifetime.

Oh, *if winter comes, can spring be far behind.* When the sun begins to shine daily in March and they know the summer break will soon be here, they know they have weathered more than a winter storm and will be able to continue their studies.

Joan's dad, Virg, begins to clear the lot and build the foundation for the home he has dreamed he will build one day. He has only Tom, his son, to help him so he practically is building it alone. In order to make some money as well as to help Virg with his ambition, Ray J. works every hour he has between classes and then all day during the summer.

Now they can laugh about it, but at the time it was scary. Sudden winds appear in that part of Colorado. One day Tom and Ray J. are on the roof trying to get the shingles nailed down. Out of the blue a big gust of wind sweeps down and picks up boards and shingles and sends them through the air. They hug that roof and hang on for dear life for at least fifteen minutes. They hear later on the radio that it blew-over twenty-eight mobile homes in a park over at Boulder.

Tom goes to Canada to study music with some professor he has met. John works out his schedule and comes to work on the house with them. Each morning at break time, Joan and her mother bring Heather and a snack to the worksite. They stop to eat and play with Heather. One day Virg is pouring cement and puts her hands in the steps. That house has changed hands several times through the years but the handprints of Heather remain in the steps leading to the outside entrance to the master bedroom. *Some memories are made in concrete to last a lifetime.*

Oklahoma

That spring is one for the birds with Joan doubling up on her course work to get that out of the way. John takes added courses to make up for the education courses he hadn't taken for his degree. Ray J. supervises student teachers (they need the money), takes orals, defends his dissertation, and Joan sends out resumes trying to find a teaching position for fall.

Everything is in place. The University assures Ray J. that he will graduate in the summer session and be a real live doctor for fall section. In desperation, he goes to the "Meat Market" in Chicago and gets several interviews but no job. Finally, he gets the invitation to be interviewed at a small university in western Oklahoma.

The position open is in the area of Reading, so Ray J. feels comfortable in the interview. He sits in the "Hot Seat" in a large room with all the members of the School of Education firing questions at him. He will be teaching in both the undergraduate division and in the graduate if he gets the position. The only courses he will be teaching in the undergraduate will be with entering freshmen; actually, one course, "Improvement of Reading".

He drives back home, feeling confident he has the position, although they had told him they would let him know later. Now he is really excited, and Joan and John are almost as excited.

Dr. Reynolds calls on Friday to congratulate him and says his contract is waiting for his signature. That is one weekend when nobody does any studying or worrying or wondering about the future. They call everybody they know to tell them the good news.

They drive down with the thought of renting a three-bedroom house but arrive late at night and have only the next day to find one in order to get back home, get their belongings, and get settled in time for opening classes.

The real estate agent, Mark, informs them that there are neither three-bedroom houses nor apartments for rent in this university town. He says he knows of a four-bedroom house they can buy, and they can look at it right now. Desperate, they walk through it, fall in love with it, and write a check for the down payment. They're back on the road to Colorado by

2PM. Mark didn't tell them until they make out the check that it is his house they just bought.

If there is a place on this earth with more beautiful people than Oklahoma, they have not found it. It is dark, they are on an unknown highway and out of gas, not knowing how far it is to the next gas station. A pickup truck suddenly stops beside them with a man and woman in it. She rolls down the window and he leans over her and asks what the problem is. Ray J. explains they are out of gas and asks if he can ride with them into a town. They both say no for they observe the pregnant woman and small child in the car. They tell Ray J. to get back in the car and lock the doors until they return with the gas. He and Joan sit in wonder until they return with the gas, put it in the gas tank, wish them well, and drive off without a penny for the gas and their trouble. *I was a stranger and you took me in.*

Such is their introduction to the Bible belt and their approach to helping a neighbor. "A days work for a days pay" is the refrain they hear from students as well as those who work in services.

Spreading Wings

In the ten years of their stay in Oklahoma, not once do they waver in their love for the people of Oklahoma. They do complain about the seventy miles to Oklahoma City that they have to drive to be in a city of any size. Their small town has only small businesses that are locally owned. Some things have to be ordered by mail or gotten from larger cities. At that time, they didn't even have a McDonalds, a Burger King, or a Kentucky Fry; sometimes an aggravation but definitely good for the kids.

Speaking of kids, John and his two kids appear to be on their way to a happier life. While John is in his last classes before graduation, he meets Gertie, a young lady who is also getting over a divorce and getting her special education certificate to teach. She has no children but seems to be fond of his two girls.

John has an interview for a position in a junior high school in Durango, and Gertie has one in elementary in Jefferson county. They each sign their contracts and feel good about finding jobs so easily. After a week of being in town looking for a place to live, John finds a small house on a fifty-foot lot not too far from school. Gertie has agreed to look after the girls while he is gone, so when he gets back and sees how happy they are together, he asks Gertie to marry him. She also has found that she is happy to be a mother of a ready-made family, so she agrees. When the Jefferson county principal agrees to let her out of her contract, they move to Durango.

What a busy year for Joan! She takes her comps, goes through orals, finishes and defends her dissertation, and has a baby.

During her pregnancy, she talks to Heather about the baby. Together, they rub her belly and tell the baby how much they love it and want it to be a part of their family. Soon, Heather is calling it her baby brother and telling him how anxious she is to have him to love. Even before his birth Derek was a welcomed addition to their family. These two have a special bond that is formed before his arrival.

October 30th their son arrives. They can hardly wait to get back to North Carolina to show him to Mother. Only three years before, they had proudly rushed back to present Heather, but this time they come prepared; they bring extra shoes. On their previous visit, on a Saturday night before their plane is to leave on Sunday, Doug's wife Lib has washed some clothes for them. No one will forget the look on her face when she comes into the den from the laundry room and announces,

"The dryer melted the soles of Heather's shoes."

She knows the manager of a department store, and when she calls him and explains what has happened, he graciously meets them downtown at 11:30 on a Saturday night and opens the store for them to buy a pair of shoes. Such is the kindness of the people of the South.

1980's

Farewell to Mother

Since her husband' death about 25 years ago, Ray J.'s mother lives with first one of her kids and then another. The past five years she has been with Doug and Lib. Every time Ray J. and family go to visit, they automatically stay with them.

They arrange to be with his mother on her birthday, August 23. Ray J. notices she is very quiet, but she looks happy, more so than usual. As they are getting the kids ready to go home, she pulls him aside so the others can't hear and says,

"Ray J., do be careful that you always do the very best that you can for your children. God has trusted them in your care, so He must think you and Joan are worthy of them. I have accomplished what God intended for me. I have seen my kids and grandkids reach the stage of life where I am no longer needed."

As they pull out of the drive, Ray J. turns to Joan,

"We won't be seeing Mother many more times in this life."

They don't get to see her again, for she has a stroke December 16 and dies within three days.

What a difference in his mother's leaving as compared to his Dad's. Ray J. cried for days after his dad's funeral, but all thirty-two kids, grandkids, and great grandkids gather back at Doug and Lib's home after his mother's funeral. They laugh and joke and talk of how much their mother would have enjoyed being with the family, sitting there quietly listening to her family enjoying themselves. What a blessing she was and is to so many people.

The very next month, which is January, Marilee has a sudden stroke and dies the next day. Poor Marilee. Just when she and Jim settle into a life that is pleasant, and they plan to retire in North Carolina, it is not to be. Anne and John fly back to North Carolina and see their mother laid to rest. So many questions with so few answers put both of them into therapy. *The hardest part of loving is learning to let go.*

Before Derek is a year old, the university hires Joan to head the Counseling Department. Now, once again, the two of them are working in the same school again, rushing home to a young, growing family. They have their evenings, weekends, and every spare moment to enjoy two very bright children growing up too quickly into being independent and going off to school. John is already teasing the young ones,

"Oh, yes, Dad will let you cross the street by yourself when you get to be about sixteen or so."

The weeks pass quickly and each semester seems to get shorter and shorter. At Christmas break they always take the time to get out of town and relax, either with Joan's parents or with John's family in Colorado.

Tornado

The word "tornado" is a frightening word until a person gets to see one up close. One afternoon Joan and Ray J. are driving over to Custer City to pick up the kids from school. They notice some dark clouds forming ahead so they think they might be in for a storm until they come over a hill and a highway patrolman stops them.

"Have you not been listening to your radio? A tornado is due here any moment. Pull off the road and turn off the motor."

They watch the clouds and see a tornado in the making. First, a small funnel dips down from the clouds and then springs back up. As the clouds grow darker, the funnel gets larger and dips lower until a large one hits the ground. Hail starts peppering their car, and the wind whistles as they watch in amazement as the tornado moves on up north. It disappears almost as suddenly as it appeared.

Friends That Last

In moving from state to state and from school to school, it is easy enough to make acquaintances, but real friends are rare. They still have Wayne and Sue, and in this town they make friends with Jeff and Cheryl who teach in their department. Their son and daughter play soccer in the same league as Heather and Derek.

They are also into country line dancing, and Oklahoma is full of the huge buildings especially built for a thousand or more to gather at one time. Practically every Friday night Ray J. and Joan get together with them to dance until late into the night. They wear typical cowboy hats and blue shirts and jeans with the stomping sounding loud and clear.

The family they meet that remains their close friends even today are Harold and Virginia who live up the hill on the street above them. Harold teaches premed courses at the university while Virginia teaches first grade in the local system. Their three daughters are close in age to Heather and Derek and they all play soccer. The two families have bonded so well through the years that they are family.

Many years after they move away, Ray J. is staying with them for a week while he supervises some repair work on some of their rental property. Joan calls one evening to tell him that she is seriously depressed when the doctor suspects a return of the cancer. The comfort of two pairs of loving arms around him as he sobs will never be forgotten.

It is some time later when they come to Durango to visit that Joan is able to thank them in person for being there for him. As usual, they bring pictures of their girls and their families and are glad to see how well Joan looks. One year, two, sometimes more, can pass without seeing one another but phone calls, cards and letters keep their ties binding.

Retirement

So many changes have been taking place at the university. Dr. Reynolds, the dean, has moved up to be the Vice President of the University and has managed to get his "good ole boy" to replace him as Dean.

The "good ole boy" approach in education just will not work. How can it, when this "good ole boy" from Texas jumps from three years as a junior high physical education teacher to the dean of a school with so many branches within it that has no professor in it with so little experience. Almost immediately the School of Education feels the downward plunge the school will have until he is finally forced out (and by a female President).

Any good leader knows to surround himself with the very best people who can fill in the areas in which he is weak. This guy is so ignorant and has so little experience to fall back on that he does the opposite. He turns down every new position for any person who is qualified and approves those who are as ignorant as he.

When Geary takes over the school, every member has a doctor's degree with the rank of professor and wide backgrounds of experiences. He begins to fill each new vacancy with instructors with masters' degrees with very little experience. One new member is a waitress in his favorite restaurant downtown.

One by one each department either crumbles entirely or becomes so weak that the reputation of the school is damaged almost beyond repair. Two years after Joan leaves, the Counseling Department is reduced to being just a few classes taught by the Psych Boys (and everyone knows what a bunch of weaklings they are).

The Reading Department takes a little longer to go under because Charlotte and Jana are still there to fight for it. The last time Ray J. has a chance to visit with Charlotte, she fills him in on how bad it got before she retired. It's almost like somebody they knew had died, so he no longer asks about it.

The last really peculiar thing Joan and Ray J. remember happening while they were still there was the hiring of the "Gay Professor", as everyone called him behind his back. When he invited Ray J. to ride with him into the city one Friday after their last class, Ray J. just assumed it was to do some shopping for things they couldn't get in town.

An hour's drive, so they chat mostly about school. Then they pull up to an apartment and he says he will be only a minute, so just sit tight. Ray J. begins to feel a little awkward when he comes back in a few minutes and introduces this guy as his lover. Ray J. hasn't been around gays when they were that blatant, so he is glad when the shopping is over and they get back home.

Some of the professors had been puzzled from the beginning when the Dean held out to hire this guy. Everyone remembered when he came back from OU one time and in a full faculty meeting told them how disgusted he was when he saw guys wearing gay T-shirts. His exact words were, "I wanted to take a knife and castrate every one of them."

Colorado

For several years Ray J. has been buying into the retirement system some of the years of his past experience. For each two years of teaching experience in another state, he can buy one year for retirement purposes. They are looking ahead to the time when the small school system where the kids are attending will not be offering the advanced classes that they want them to have.

One summer while visiting the family in Durango, they find just the place they think is almost perfect. They make a down payment on in.

In October, Ray J. turns in his papers for early retirement for the following June 30th. They decide to retire in Durango where they will be close enough to see family from both sides. Ray J. had missed knowing his grandparents, only Granny until he was 10, so he wants their kids to know at least one complete set of grandparents.

They work for three months clearing the huge front and back yards. The pasture has so many fruit trees covered with small trees that they don't realize some of them are there. The house had been built in three stages so it looks OK. They decide to get the outside more presentable and then tackle the inside. They throw many of their small items into a long tack room that runs across most of the house in back. The three bedrooms and bath upstairs had been the last stage built so there are closets galore in all three rooms, even running together in the low eves of the south side. The kids cram them full and close the doors.

A three-car garage is not attached to the house but it's almost new and airtight. It is easy to store extra furniture and piles of boxes in it and let the cars sit outside until winter comes when they will have nothing better to do than put things away.

Heather and Derek are excited about being in the same school system with Lisa and Rachael at the high school with Heather and Derek at the junior high where John is teaching. They begin to get anxious about getting their clothes ready for school so they leave the outside work and start in the house.

House of Mystery

Cleaning out the tack room is quite a chore, but they plan to buy a couple of horses for riding and the tack room will be put to good use. They know the house has a basement or a cellar, so when Joan finds a trap door in the middle of the room, she opens it.

"Wow! Come look at this. There is a cistern standing full of water down there."

She quickly closes that and moves on into the laundry room. Here she finds another trap door with stairs that go down into a damp cellar, so they close that and put the dryer over the door.

Later, as Joan is making up the bed in their bedroom room upstairs, a telephone keeps ringing, but the phone is dead each time she lifts the receiver. When it continues to ring, she opens the closet door and discovers a ringing phone just inside the closet. When she lifts the receiver, a voice says,

"Who is speaking, please?"

"This is Joan Pharr. Who are you and how did you get this number?"

"Hi. This is Joyce and I live next door, next to your pasture. I will be right over."

In just a few minutes, the doorbell rings and both Joan and Ray J. are there to answer it, anxious to find out what mystery lies ahead. They invite Joyce into the living room and listen in awe and a little frightened as she tells the history of the house they have bought and the one she and her husband bought just a few months ago.

"A few years back, a woman and two men made the headlines when they tried to extort fifteen million dollars from Gulf Oil Company. Our house and yours could have been the scene of a movie one night when the

FBI surround the places and the lights are as bright as day. A deep voice over a foghorn shouts (just like the movies),

'You are surrounded. Come out with your arms raised high above your head.'

"A man from your house (not yours at the moment of course) walks out with his arms over his head and peacefully surrenders. A man and a woman come from ours and give no trouble as the officers take them away. Everyone in the valley had wondered who the mysterious couple and their companion next door were and why they rarely spoke to anyone else.

"When they appeared out of nowhere and bought the two places for cash, there was speculation that they might be connected to the robbery of the gold that was stolen from the Silverton Mine Company. Now that they knew they had plotted the extortion ever since they came here, your place has been searched with a fine toothcomb but no gold was found.

"Soon after we bought and moved in, I was in an upstairs bedroom cleaning out a closet when I found a large grocery bag full of hand grenades. That same closet had the phone that was connected to your house, so this is how the two groups communicated with each other in their plotting."

This information gets Ray J. and Joan starting to look at their place a little differently. Maybe the gold is buried in the cistern under the tack room? What about that old run-down cellar out by the garage or that large mound out in the pasture? Oh, it could be buried anywhere.

That happened years ago and the FBI and several other agencies have searched this place with modern equipment so it surely isn't here, or they would have found it. Oh, well. They often muse aloud with "What if?"

They have the cistern filled in with rock and dirt and seal off the trap door. John knows a young man who is a jack-leg carpenter. He does an excellent job with paneling the room with aspen. Joan and Ray J. do the carpet and paint the facing around the door and windows. Now they have a beautiful den where they can sit on the couch and look out toward the mountains in back.

Together, they buy the lumber and build a chicken house. The kids have such fun watching the twenty-five little biddies grow into full-grown chickens. Growing up on a farm, killing a chicken, picking its feathers, and cutting it up to eat is just a natural process, but Joan takes the kids and makes some excuse to go into town every time Ray J. tells her that he is going to kill another chicken.

Soon, they are down to one rooster and fourteen hens. Ray J. stands in amazement to see Joan as excited as the kids when they gather their first eggs.

"Hey, Ray J. How many eggs does a hen lay at one time? Do they lay every day?

"What is so unusual about fresh eggs in a nest and you gathering them? I guess I must have gathered thousands of them when I was a kid."

Ray J. forgets at times that Joan didn't grow up on a farm and know all these things. She doesn't even know the difference between straw and hay, so he tells her.

"Straw is the stalk from wheat or grain of any kind and is used for bedding; it has no food value. Hay is the grass, clover, alfalfa, or other vegetation with food value put into bales to be fed during the winter months when there is no green grass for the horses and cows to eat."

Anne Returns

Anne and her luck with men! Her next attempt at happiness with a man looks favorable for a few years. This time, she has gone in the opposite direction and living in the lap of luxury: private plane to take them anywhere she wants (now her dog, Flapper, can go since she refused to let him ride commercial and be put in a cage), buy any type clothes, furniture, or car she desires. Yet, she isn't a happy person and begins to have headaches, upset stomach, even hospitalized at one point, but they find nothing wrong.

John has just recently bought a 4-acre place with plenty of room, so when Anne calls and says, "Please come get me before I lose my mind", he goes after her immediately. It will be weeks before she fully recovers, but surrounded with love and attention, she comes to realize that her problem is not a physical but a psychological one. Although she had money, she did not have the attention she needs.

When she first moved to California, she had started with a bank as a teller. They sent her to workshops and various training sessions until she became an officer of the bank. Once on her feet and feeling good again, she has little trouble finding a position as an assistant to the personnel officer in a local bank, and soon moves up to his position when he gets booted up.

Alternative School

Ray J. cannot handle retirement because he is bored and needing something to do the minute they finish cleaning up the yard and pasture. Discovering that the school district has been searching for years to find the right person to organize and direct an alternative school, he makes an appointment and goes in to see the Superintendent of Schools.

They talk for hours about the drug problem in Durango, the many wealthy families who come here to play and just let their kids run wild, the extreme wealth and the very poor with few in between.

Ray J. tells him his ideas about the selections of students, the guide lines they will follow, how to handle PE and advanced sciences in regular classes, and so forth. The Superintendent likes his ideas so well that he is put on the agenda for the next board meeting which is the next Tuesday night. He is the first on the agenda and in just a few minutes after he presents his ideas, they approve and say they will give him a contract.

Who would have believed a whole new life will open for Ray J. and Joan. An Alternative School within a school opens that fall in one of the reading rooms of the library. Twelve students have been approved for the program with the understanding that Ray J. has complete charge of their lives. They have to report to him by 8 AM each morning of the week, attend five classes, some with him and others in the regular classes, and then be on the job of his selection and work for at least four hours a day. They sign contracts that state that any violation will automatically put them out of the school.

Durango is a tourist town, so Ray J. has little difficulty in finding jobs for them when he explains the program at a business club meeting. Employers are happy to hire part time students when they know the teacher has control and they cannot just walk off the job.

Joan continues to work in the yard planting flowers, putting out rose bushes, and keeping the grass cut. When Ray J. takes on the job of being the director of the alternative school, she takes over most of the work around the house.

Her background in psychology and counseling plus her experiences help the program far more than anyone else knows. They sometimes laugh and sometimes cry when Ray J. brings home actual stories of the students in the program.

Most of the students who come into the program have been into drugs, sex, theft, and other minor crimes. Whenever one of them gets caught shop lifting or for being drunk, or on drugs, they always give Ray J.'s phone number and the officer calls day or night, mostly night, and mostly after 2 AM. Off he goes to put up bail in the early days, and as the police grow to know and trust him, give his word the kid will appear in court or do whatever is needed. As time passes and the kids develop more trust in Ray J. to do what is best for them, these incidents become fewer and fewer.

One day the officers bring into the school a little girl who has been sitting on a rock high above the river for at least sixteen days. They have become concerned about her mental state. Thinking she has no one, Ray J. takes her into the program and tell kids to help her get settled into school and working. Soon they are telling him some pretty tall tales she is telling them, but he pays no attention.

She finishes the school year and comes back the following fall. Ray J. is encouraged to think she is getting into a normal life. One day a detective appears, shows his credentials, and tells the background of this so-called orphan. In reality, she is the granddaughter of a very wealthy California woman who has hired detectives on several occasions to find her. Several years ago, this lady has given the inheritance their father left them to her two sons, one of whom was the father of the girl in question. He takes the money and soon spends it on building a "show-case" of a house, and then the remainder on gambling and drugs. At one point he has sold her to a group of traveling gypsies, and it takes three months to find her and buy her back. She has been telling the truth all along when she told the kids she would inherit three million dollars when she reaches twenty-one.

Randy is the one who comes so close to being thrown out of the program. He is such a hyperactive kid of fifteen. Ray J. can handle his using his knees to make the table dance and the kids complaining, but his barnyard language is more than he can permit in a class setting. He calls him "My cross to bear" so many times, the kids start referring to him as "My Cross-Eyed Bear".

Checking on the three students that he has working at the Durango Chocolate Factory, Ray J. comments to the supervisor how difficult it is to place someone who is hyperactive. The lady says she can use someone like that in making chocolate patties.

The next Friday when Ray J. goes out to check on him, he walks into the workroom and finds Randy sitting at a long table with several other employees. He is taking a ball of chocolate and gleefully patting it into a chocolate patty. The lady in charge said Randy did more patties in his four-hour shift than most of the others did in their eight.

The whole town knew about Megan and her sister when their family blew into town. They had just sold their shopping center in Michigan and have more money than Midas. Reaching the age of forty with absolutely no reason to work, they arrive in town, buy matching jeeps and give the kids their own bank account and set them free. If ever there was an accident waiting to happen, these two are willing souls.

Megan is suspended almost immediately from high school when they catch her passing "joints" in the hall, trying to buy new friends. Her sister is caught soon after, doing the same stunt at the junior high. Megan is far too intelligent to be satisfied with doing drugs and hanging out with the "less than bright" kids on the street. Ray J. takes her into the program and treats her the same as the others. She knows if she doesn't conform to the rules and regulations, she will be back out on the streets.

Very quickly she lets the other kids know she is wealthy and not accustomed to being bossed around and having to work. Ray J. decides to let the kids handle her attitude and see if things won't work out. One morning she complains in a loud voice,

"Dr. Pharr, make them quit calling me a bitch."

"Quit acting like one and I will," is the quick answer he gives her. Beginning with that incident, Megan changes her attitude and settles into working very hard both in her studies and in her work.

She becomes seventeen by the end of the school year. Ray J. calls her into his office and has a long discussion with her about her future. She has grown to respect him and knows that he has her best interest at heart. When he explains that she is eligible to take the GED, skip the rest of high school, and get into college next fall, she hugs him and says she will be forever grateful.

Three years later, she proves he was right when she walks in and tells everyone that she used to be in this program and is now a college graduate. She has gone to school in straight semesters, including summers.

In his eight years of being the Director of the Alternative School, which expanded and moved to its own location with more students and teachers, the percentage of the students who went on to higher education was far greater than those in the regular school system. These years of working in this setting are the most rewarding of his teaching career.

Farewell to Virg

Few things remain constant; such is life. Here Ray J. and Joan have moved to Colorado to be near family, and for a few years they have gained so much from being close to the grandkids, watching them grow along with their two kids, and finally Virg and Corinne are driving down from Loveland to see them on a regular basis. The long evenings by the fire playing bridge with nothing to interfere for the whole weekend are the most enjoyable times they have ever had with them.

The telephone call comes one early morning about 4AM, awakening them from a deep sleep. Joan answers the phone as she always sleeps on the side of the bed where the phone is. Ray J. knows from the catch in her voice as she says, "Oh, no," that something has to be wrong, and then she

says, "I'll be there as quickly as I can get a plane out of here," and she
drops the phone and flings herself on top of him sobbing,

"Oh, darling, Dad had a heart attack and he's in the hospital."

As Ray J. calls the airport and makes the arrangements for her to leave
immediately, she throws a few things in an overnight. Luckily the airport
is so small and the planes are too so it is easy to catch a short flight to Denver. Before they can get out of the house and into the car, the phone rings
again and it is her cousin Bill calling,

"Oh, Ray J. I hate to tell you, but Virg just died."

They leave the kids asleep upstairs as he rushes her to catch the flight. It
is obvious Joan is in shock as she walks out to the plane like a zombie. Ray
J. can do nothing more for her and he needs to get back to the house
before the kids awaken and wonder where they are.

It is late afternoon before Joan calls back to give the particulars. The
doctors tell them while lying there with them working so hard to save his
life, Virg had looked up at them and said,

"You are working awfully hard. It's ok. I've lived a good life and I'm
ready to go home." With that said, he closes his eyes and dies.

That special bond that binds father and daughter brings Joan to her
knees in prayer, so grateful for the years she had him to share in finding
herself and for him to know she has found what she wanted out of life. *The
hardest part of loving is learning to let go.*

Cancer One

Within two years, they are in a battle like none they ever dreamed would
happen. There is no history of any women in her family having such a
thing. Joan discovers a lump in her right breast and goes immediately for a
mammogram. The exam shows nothing, but determined to find out why
the lump and its continued growth, she goes in for a biopsy. This, too,
shows nothing, but the doctor is a friend and he performs a fine needle
aspiration which saves Joan's life. A very fine doctor removes her right
breast along with all the lymph nodes; in other words, a radical.

While still heavy with sedation, Joan cannot believe the oncologist when he says,

"I have just seen the fastest growing cancer I have ever seen removed from your breast. Five years is what we usually give the patient with cancer, but I suggest you make your plans even shorter."

Putting together the strongest chemotherapy drugs they have devised thus far, the doctors begin the weekly treatments. With eyes closed and her hands in Ray J.'s, she visualizes the drugs as little creatures running through her veins to catch the cancer cells and destroy them. He carries her home, semi asleep, semi drugged, and puts her to bed downstairs in the guest bedroom where he spends the night beside her.

The six weeks of treatment are finally over. With only a few days rest, she next begins the radiation treatments. How exhausted she is after each, and they wait and pray for the treatments to be over. That day finally arrives when all the treatments are over with the scars and burns from them to be a reminder forever. Ironically, before this awful disaster, she has never given any thought of dying, like most people, but this forces her to look at the possibility and come to peace with it. *O Death, Where is thy sting. O Grave. Where is thy victory?*

Once it is evident that Joan is out of immediate danger, the good humor and the teasing come back into play. Joan is completely bald and walks around slightly one-sided with only one breast. She has ordered a "boob" as they will always call it, but it hasn't arrived as yet. Derek puts a tennis ball in his shirt only on one side and walks around asking if they think he looks a lot like Mom.

One day he brings a friend home and introduces him to his mother,

"Ryan, have you met my bald headed, lop-sided mother?"

With a death in the family and a near death, they maintain a positive outlook on life and laugh at the events that threatened them. Reading Norman Cousins' works will remain with them for they believe he had the right attitude about the humor in healing. Joan and Ray J. carry cards that have the following for anyone who is associated with cancer:

Cancer is so limited…
It cannot cripple love,

It cannot shatter hope,
It cannot corrode Faith,
It cannot eat away at peace,
It cannot destroy confidence,
It cannot kill friendship,
It cannot shut out memories,
It cannot silence courage,
It cannot invade the soul,
It cannot reduce eternal life,
It cannot quench the spirit,
It cannot lessen the power of resurrection,
Remember: Disease is not our problem.
Our problem is despair.

Before too long, the routine of life begins. Joan still shows up religiously at the volleyball games, wearing a large sock in her bra until the boob arrives, and wearing a different cover on her head until she can find a wig that will stay on and yet not be too tight.

John has been the coach long enough to build a great reputation, even among other coaches throughout the state. His team has gone to State twelve times out of the last thirteen and has won State eleven of those. Lisa, Rachael, and Heather all play on first string. Ray J. is one of the scorekeepers at every home game, Derek is one of the loudest cheerleaders from the crowd, and Joan, Anne, (sometimes Gertie) are stomping their feet at every point.

Joan didn't know she has so many friends until she comes to the first game after being away so long. Seems about half the crowd that night comes over to say something to her.

When Lisa graduates from high school, she enters a liberal arts college in Denver that has a strong art program. The family is greatly relieved that she is that close to home; they were afraid she would move to some "artsy" place and go to some college that wasn't even accredited.

1990's

Anne meets a college instructor when she takes a business course and within the year she marries him. He moves into her small house with her.

Just when they think that *Life can be beautiful* again, John shows up at their door with a black eye and bruises on his face and confesses to an awful truth they are in shock to hear. For years Gertie has been abusing him when she loses her temper, but now she has begun to abuse the girls. Twice he has walked into the house and caught her on the floor on top of Lisa. Last night she has Rachael on the floor, and when he pulls her off, she turns on him and hits him with the poker from the fireplace.

Now, they all have the problem with what to do about it. It is easy enough to help John and Rachael move in with them for the time being, but it is against the law to know about an abuser, especially a teacher, and not report it. If they do report it, she loses her license to teach anywhere in the state and maybe just anywhere, but if they don't report it, both John and Ray J. could lose theirs.

Even though she has been abusing him for years, John just cannot agree to doing that to her. Ray J. and Joan can afford to chance it because he doesn't have to teach, but John gambles everything if he is discovered covering for her. The whole family, including Anne and her new husband, get together and agree it will be a very quiet divorce with no one revealing this secret.

New Mexico

The following year Heather graduates and enters UNC as a freshman. What a void in their lives with both Lisa and Heather gone, but luckily they are in Colorado and can fly or drive home any weekend.

Starting in the spring, John turns in his resignation, gets accepted into the doctoral program of NMSU in Las Cruces, New Mexico, and Heather puts in a transfer to the same school. Of course it is no surprise when Rachael graduates in June and applies to the same school.

After a year, John realizes he cannot continue with his studies and at the same time support two daughters in college, so they move to Southern

California. He goes back into teaching in a high school and his girls transfer to the state college system.

Ray J. retires and they move to Las Cruces, New Mexico. With furniture packed in two large trucks, Joan drives one and Ray J. the other; they begin a new life. Moving into a three bedroom, two-bath home with a small swimming pool, they feel they are alone after all these years and now the quiet years of their lives will begin.

Cancer Two

Two years and three months later, during a routine physical checkup, the doctor finds a small lump during a prostate examination on Ray J. He makes the arrangements to do a biopsy December 14th at the local hospital.

In a very short time, the doctor's nurse calls and says the doctor wants him to see him at once. He goes in that afternoon for they have been anxious to get the results. For once in his life, he doesn't have to wait as his nurse takes him into the doctor's office.

"Just as I suspected, it is malignant and I've already made the arrangements with the hospital for we don't want to wait any longer to cut it out."

He becomes angry with Ray J. when he tells him he wants a second opinion.

"I know the other three urologists in town, and they will all agree with me. It should be cut out as soon as possible. You are only wasting time."

Although somewhat experimental, Cryosurgery seems to be the latest procedure. Joan searches and researches to find out more about it, but there isn't much to find out except how expensive it is.

She finds there are four hospitals that have the expensive equipment. The two that are west of the Mississippi are in Denver and San Diego. They debate about which is closer and which is easier to drive. San Diego is straight out west on I 10 and then I 8, and Denver is straight up north on I 25. Since it is winter and the mountains to climb to Denver could prove dangerous, they investigate San Diego. They quickly change their minds when they find that the best-known urologist in the country, Dr. David Lawford, performs the procedure at University Hospital in Denver.

Since his PSA was really high and the biopsy has proven to be malignant, the doctor schedules the operation in two days so Joan and Ray J. decide to remain in the motel and not return home until after the operation.

When Ray J. awakens, Joan says everything went well according to the nurses, but she hasn't had a chance to talk to David. A very young doctor comes in later and says he is the follow-up, for Dr. Lawford is now in Sweden and his tour of lectures won't be over for another three months.

When the oncologist comes in and starts with "And what are your five-year plans," Joan and Ray J. burst out laughing and ask him to leave. Frank, the follow-up doctor, inquires about their refusal to see the oncologist, and they tell him they don't need him so just explain what the next steps will be.

Seems like only yesterday they sat and waited to hear the news of cancer, as Joan takes his hand and they listen to Frank.

Insurance has become the ruler of their lives, and it rules that he must be out of the hospital several days before the tubes come out. He has one in his penis, his belly, and an incision just below the penis: one for the freezing process, one for the heating of vital organs, and one for the withdrawal of tissue. An attendant helps him to the car and they stay in a motel for it is very late at night by now.

Neither one is able to sleep, so they pack their bags and leave the motel by the time the sun comes up. Barely out of the city and Ray J. begins to vomit, black out, vomit again, and then repeat. Joan pulls off the interstate at the first stop, and Ray J. lies down on a bench to make the world stop turning. Every time he stands up, he vomits some more until finally there is nothing but green bile. He crawls into the car and tells Joan,

"Just get me home and let me die in my own bed."

Joan, ever the careful driver with never a speeding ticket, refuses to look at the speedometer as she flies down the freeway. In the years to come they laugh and they cry about this wild night of terror. *How do I love thee? Let me count the ways.*

To be in a city seven hundred miles from the hospital where the surgery was performed is a little frightening until all three urologists in town say,

"No way! You had experimental surgery under the government's supervision, so I'm not about to touch you. I'm not setting myself up for a law suit that my insurance won't cover."

Panic sets in because the tubes need to be removed within so many days or complications will set in. Calling every urologist in the southwest, Joan finally finds one over in El Paso who says,

"Bring him over and I'll yank them out".

Only a urologist with the name "Dr. Dicky" has the nerve to do the job. When the tubes are out and Ray J. has calmed down, he explains how wrong the doctors are who think no one but a government doctor would ever touch him. The procedure was an experimental one but not under the government.

And now almost a year passes with Joan working full time at the community college while Ray J. mopes around the house wearing old clothes and wetting his pants. He reads those articles where men have killed the doctors for leaving them this way, but this is better than the alternative. The operation was successful. All he has to do is to watch the tissue flow out with the urine, but he has little control over his bladder.

Summer comes and with it comes John, for his school is out. What a surprise to hear his son, the teacher, the minister, say,

"Dad, get the hell of the house and go to work. All of us are tired of seeing you this way."

With the shock of that remark, Joan jumps into the conversation with,

"I cannot believe my own ears. You have never said such a harsh thing to anybody, and now to say it to your dad! I am truly shocked!"

"Shock" is what he is after. He has investigated the treatment for incontinence through his doctor in California. There are several types of medication now on the market for help in living with this condition.

Texas

Life can be beautiful once again. To think that such small pills can do wonders in controlling his bladder is almost beyond him. With only a small plastic sac to catch any sudden surprises, he now wears regular clothes and is anxious to go to work.

A friend of Joan's suggests a complete change of lifestyles may be the answer.

"Why not buy a franchise for a Burger King or KFC or something that will make some money. Don't you think it's time you two get out of the helping profession and help yourselves for a change?"

That question brings on a healthy laugh from both of them. As if they needed the money or that they haven't been helping themselves all their lives by teaching. As John has said many times,

"Dad, let's face it. We have that teacher mentality about money. If only we can make enough to stay off the welfare rolls, why ask for more?"

Waco, not Wacho

The idea of a change of lifestyle does sound appealing so Joan and her secretary start researching franchises, looking for one that does a service rather than just making money. Direct Marketing is nationwide with a franchise in any city of a size that appeals to them. They find one for sale in Waco, Texas, and Joan has a lawyer check out its credibility.

Feeling secure, they fill out all the papers they require and send them into the company's headquarters in Florida. They can't believe it, but a man flies out from Dallas as a representative of the company to interview them. Now they are really impressed and can hardly wait for an answer to their application.

They sign a contract which requires them to begin the work at once which creates a problem. Joan has another year to finish out her contract with the community college. For the first time in their married life, they will be separated for more than a week. Ray J. packs his things and moves to Texas and leaves Joan behind in New Mexico. He rents a living room kitchen combination with a bedroom and bath in an apartment complex and spends his nights on the phone talking with Joan.

The next year is the most frustrating, the most difficult, and the most exciting one he experiences in a long time. He spends long hours learning the business (so much paper work to plow through during the long evening hours) and how to become a salesman while Joan travels across the southwest expanding the program she is developing for the community colleges throughout the state. They spend a fortune in telephone bills calling every night.

It is true there have been *Innocents Abroad,* but none quite so innocent as Ray J. and Joan when it comes to the business world. The mother company that owns the Direct Marketing Company is, indeed, a reputable one, but the ones selling the franchise are not *the pure in heart.* Too late, hey discover the previous owners of this franchise had taken the business-men's money and left town without mailing the advertisements. In fact, they have been caught and are serving time in prison.

Joan drives over from Las Cruces, and they ponder their situation for days. Believing in the basic goodness of mankind and having read *In His Steps,* they decide to invest even further into the business. They give free advertising to those who have invested and gotten nothing for their money. They no longer require written contracts.

Living in the Bible belt, the customers understand when they say, "We are following in the footsteps of One who once walked among us, and a handshake is all we ask." Very few people take advantage and refuse to pay for their advertising once they have it mailed. The others soon spread the word about them and business increases rather quickly.

Next summer seems so far away as Joan goes back to finish out her contract, and Ray J. works on alone. One evening John calls to tell him that when his school is out, he plans to help him during the whole month of July. Good news; bad news. Good, that he will be with him that month and then in August Joan will be moving their things over, never to live apart again. Bad, that now he has to find better living quarters.

They had sold the house in California, which gives Ray J. his GI Bill to buy a house again. Now he uses every day between eleven and one to look for houses. During the lunch hour is not the time to try to sell business-men anything but food. It must be his guardian angel to that leads him take a side street in leaving the mall one day because he finds a house for sell by owner.

Located next to a corner, the lot is pie-shaped with the backyard fenced and two shade trees in the front, but the house was built with them in mind, even though it was built thirty-eight years before.

The owner, now retired, had been a builder so he had the entry way with double doors to the left going into the living room and dining room combination, then back to the kitchen and dinette. The other door opens into a den with a door to the left going into the kitchen; another door to the right goes down a hall to the master bedroom and bath on the left and two bedrooms and bath on the right. There are double doors straight in front that open into his office, which is huge. One wall has a built-in desk and drawers and shelves to keep everything out of sight. A door to the right goes out into the backyard, and the one to the left opens into a dou-ble-car garage. All of this built on a slab without a single step going up or down.

Ray J. wonders why would any sane person want to sell this spacious home. Their son from Ft. Worth had been coming down on weekends to check on them and finally asked them to sell and move in with him and his wife. They are in their eighties and know it is for the best so they agree. When he tells Ray J. the price he wants, Ray J. doesn't haggle for one minute. He writes out a check for the earnest money and signs a contract.

When John arrives, they walk the streets selling direct marketing adver-tising. During the long lunch periods and late into the night, they have many long long talks about their lives and the similarities between them.

John tells him that soon after he arrived in California with the girls, he finally meets his soul mate. Her name is Paula so they call her Paula Two. She, like Joan, has never been married but older than Joan when Ray J. married her. Again, she is like Joan in wanting to marry him and help see his girls through college. So similar to Joan in many ways but more so than they ever wanted it to be as they discover about ten years later.

Paula Two's parents live in Texas just seventy miles east of Dallas in a small farming community. A few days before he must leave for home, John takes his dad to visit them.

Educated, refined, so gentle in nature, Winnie and Earl open their arms and home to them when they arrive. The men play golf most of the day while Winnie insists she stay home and have a solid meal for them in the evenings.

The first night as they are having coffee after a huge meal, Winnie asks,

"Anyone for a game of dominoes? Scratch? Forty-two? Pick your favorite."

"You mean you can play actual games with dominoes?" Ray J. asks.

"Aren't you from Waco, the domino capitol of the world?"

Both Winnie and Earl are surprised that he doesn't know that much about Waco.

"Before coming here, the only thing I know about Waco is that the Davidian Compound is in Waco and made world news with its horror of fire and death, especially of all the little innocent children. And people living there don't even talk about that."

"No wonder they don't. The Davidian Compound isn't even in Waco. It's about forty miles south on Highway 36 going toward Houston. I doubt half the people in Waco have ever been by it."

Ray J. tells them he will begin to learn more about the city when Joan comes over and his life isn't quite so hectic.

All good things must come to an end, and so does John's visit. Ray J. rides with him to Las Cruces where they rent two trucks and get their belongings packed in time for him to go home to California and Joan and Ray J. to move their things to Waco.

With Joan at home in the office to do the paper work and answer the phone, their days settle into a normal pattern. Monday through Friday, up at six with a cup of coffee and a piece of toast or a bowl of cold cereal, both of them meet appointments with owners or managers of restaurants and coffee houses. Usually another cup of coffee or tea as they sit explaining their service before the crowd comes in. From nine to eleven are the best hours for downtown businesses before the manager goes to lunch. Then back home to wait until after two when they can finish the day.

Saturdays are light days with few appointments so they explore the city and look for new stores opening or the signs of new business. Saturday and Sunday afternoons are the best times of the week, for they relax and see the beauties of the city.

In addition to being the domino capitol of the world, Waco is also the home of Dr. Pepper. They visit the Dr. Pepper Museum and learn how a local druggist started a unique-tasting soft drink of the century. The old part of downtown Waco was almost wiped out by a tornado years ago and is just now being slowly rebuilt. One of the most beautiful parks in the area is just minutes from the downtown area, extending for miles past the city zoo and spread out by the lake.

Cancer Three

For nine years they pay the high premiums for health insurance. The insurance company assures them it will be greatly reduced if Joan lives cancer free for ten years. Joan has followed her doctor's requests and gone in for her routine check-ups: every three months for years, then every four, and then six. The days before each one have been difficult for her, not knowing the outcome. Only those who live with cancer know the exact feelings that people experience during these days. With only five months to go to finish her ten years, the doctor discovers a lump in Joan's remaining breast.

As Ray J. is ready to leave for an appointment to make a sale, she bursts through the door,

"I can't! I won't! I won't go through this again! Oh, God! How can we live this way?"

He grabs her and holds her close as she sobs uncontrollably. He withdraws from his shirt pocket one of the cards they carry,

"Cancer is so limited, it cannot cripple love, it cannot shatter hope, it cannot corrode Faith…"

Finally, she settles down and says, "OK, Damn it! I will do what I have to do!"

When they see the surgeon, he says he will put her to sleep to do the biopsy, and they should decide beforehand what course they want to take. If it proves malignant, what should he do? Wake her up and discuss it, remove that portion of the breast, or remove the total breast? Without hesitation and in unison, they say,

"Remove the total breast."

It is 8:30 PM when they wheel her back from recovery and put her in a private room. Ray J. stretches out on the bed the nurse brings in and waits for her to awaken. At 4 AM, the night nurse, Petra, comes in and says,

"Mr. Pharr, it is time we get her on her feet and into the bathroom."

With Petra on one side and Ray J. on the other, they start toward the bathroom. Joan takes two steps and slumps to the floor in a dead faint. Petra gets her awake and they start again. Once again, she faints and slumps to the floor. What a sense of humor Petra has when she awakens her again and says,

"Why don't you just butt-scoot to the bathroom, and then we will sit you on the throne."

By the time she sits long enough to accomplish her mission, Joan is able to walk back to her bed with assistance.

They are learning (the hard way) that there are so many different kinds of cancer, even those in the breast. This one is nothing like the first one. Petra says,

"They just snipped it off and sewed you back up, good as new except a few pounds lighter."

Time-Out for Depression

One morning, several months after the operation, Joan doesn't get up at her usual time. Ray J. lets her sleep in because he knows she requires more sleep than he. He discovered long ago that he is a high-energy person and needs very little sleep while she is low energy and sometimes needs eight or more hours per night. He gets concerned so he takes her a glass of orange juice (she cannot live without it) and awakens her. He asks why the sleepy head this morning, and she says,

"I don't understand it. For the past several mornings I haven't felt well. It's a struggle for me to get out of bed. After you leave to make your rounds, I find myself weeping and feeling so sad. At times so overwhelming that I feel emotionally and physically drained. What do you suppose is the matter with me?"

"I don't know, but let's get you an appointment to see a doctor right away."

In a few days, she gets in to see a general practioner who prescribes Prozac and counseling. Joan chooses to skip the Prozac but does get in to see the counselor, Dee. After several sessions with the warm, British counselor, Dee decides her depression is caused by a chemical imbalance, which Joan agrees with, almost with relief, for this came about because of the chemotherapy treatments. This, in turn, brought about an early menopause, which brings a reduction in her production of estrogen.

This goes around in circles because she can't take estrogen replacement therapy, and on it goes. Dee next refers her to a psychiatrist who puts her on antidepressant therapy.

So many people think depression affects women only. The truth is that men are affected also, but few of them admit it. Most cases have been successfully treated with just a small pill to be taken daily.

Corinne

Virg and Corinne traveled a great deal during the last few years of his life, taking several cruises to Alaska, through the Panama Canal, Europe, so many she lost track of them. Since his death, she pays Joan's fare so she will go with her from time to time. They try to get Ray J to go, but his years in the Navy did the ocean thing for him.

In between the cruises, Joan runs up to see her and so do Heather and Derek. Corinne loves to have Heather visit for they go out to eat and shop. Derek goes to visit because he loves his grandmother, but he also knows there are some things around the house she loves to have him do: the furniture has to be moved from time to time. What is a woman to do in her spare time if she can't think about how the room would look if this is moved here and that is moved over there. And the light bulbs too high for her to reach just will burn out from time to time. And, then, of course, he takes his grandmother out to eat.

Joan stays home all day while she is recovering from the operation, and Ray J. goes out alone. For several weeks she keeps telling him that her mother must be staying home a lot more than usual because she calls at such odd times during the day and usually asks what time it is. He teases,

"Tell your mother it is cheaper to buy a watch than pay long distance telephoning."

Corinne's closest friend, Carmel, calls Joan one Friday morning and tells her that she should pay a surprise visit to see Corinne and see what is going on.

"Every time I visit her, the kitchen is full of groceries on the counters. I ask why she buys so many groceries when she never cooks; she always eats out. She says she forgets to take her grocery list so she buys what she thinks she needs and then finds she doesn't need them."

"None of our P.E.O. sisters will ride with her anymore. We are afraid to. One day she stops right in the middle of Lincoln Avenue and mutters 'I believe I left the iron on'."

"You know she never drives out Highway 34 that goes up to Estes Park. Yesterday, for some strange reason, she takes off up that winding, dangerous highway and winds up in Estes Park. She calls me, almost frantic, and asks for directions on how to get back home."

Joan catches the next flight available and flies up to see her. It is obvious the moment she gets there that something is wrong. The garage door is standing wide open, and anyone can walk into her house from there, which Joan does. Her mother isn't even surprised to see her.

The physical changes she sees in her mother are profound. She has gained a lot of weight and she looks a mess: matted hair, dirty old dress, and her eyes are almost glazed. The kitchen is unreal: every counter stacked high with groceries and when she opens a door, every shelf is full.

The refrigerator is full of stale, left-over meals and meat that is almost black.

Joan packs as much of her mother's clothes as she can get into her Buick and brings her back home to live. Joan laughs as she says how many times her mother asks why Joan is driving when the Buick is hers.

Joan and Ray J. move into the guest bedroom so Corinne can have theirs. She needs the walk-in closet, the walk-in shower and to be removed from the noises of the street because she is afraid of the dark and the noises.

Corinne is forever repeating herself, forgetting the time of day, the week, the month, and even the year. How frustrating it must be for her when every noise must be someone in the house looking for her. In the evenings she sees her reflection in the window and swears it's a man outside looking in at her. Joan closes the blinds and assures her she is safe with them.

"Three Coins in the Fountain"
is better than
Three Pins in a Hip

It is October 23rd, Ray J.'s birthday, when he gets up during the night to go to the bathroom. Still not accustomed to going down the hall to the guest bathroom and forgetting they have moved a small table into the hall, he stumbles over it and hits the door facing. *Oh, Dante, is this the Purgatory you saw?* His screams bring Joan running; she straightens his legs enough that he can breathe again.

"I'm going to be ok. I must have a muscle twisted for the pain is easing. Let me rest a little. You go on back to bed."

She is determined that he shall not move because he might do some serious damage. He finally agrees, so she calls for an ambulance. They are surprised how quickly it arrives. Ray J. grits his teeth as they put him on a board and wrap him with tape so firmly he cannot move a muscle.

Joan slips into some clothes (doesn't even take time to insert her "boobs") and follows them to the hospital. Rushing to go to the emergency room, an administrator stops her for insurance information. Exasperated, she digs into her purse to satisfy him.

"Oh, how we live and die by the insurance companies of America, and we even pay them for their control!"

She finally gets to see the doctor on duty who shows her his x-rays.

"It looks like he may need a hip replaced. The surgeon will know for sure when he gets into that area."

Joan stays in the face of any personnel who come her way for she wants them to know about his allergies. And now she sits and waits.

Hours later, when Ray J. is in the recovery room, she finds they didn't have to replace his hip; instead, they put three pens in it. Oh, the joys of going through airport securities with his arms held high while someone searches him and the crowd looks on. More often than not, Joan turns to the crowd with,

"I had no idea he was carrying a gun."

By early afternoon, Ray J. awakes with three pins in his right hip where it was broken, and the therapist beside the bed telling him,

"Sir, it is time for you to be awake and take a step or two."

Ray J. surprises himself when he eases out of the bed, and holding onto the walker, takes a step. Joan is with him when the nurse comes in to check, and to everyone's surprise, it is Petra. How kind and cheerful the nurses are as they help him through a surprisingly quick recovery.

As he had done for her, Joan now spends the night in the bed alongside him. Petra remembers that Joan must have her orange juice and coffee but not before she has fifteen minutes after her morning pill.

The day is cloudy with a few showers so it looks like a long day for them. Joan goes to the chapel to say her morning prayers. As she starts to leave, a ray of sunshine breaks through the skylight in the chapel, a "Godly nudge" not to worry about Ray J. What a happy note to leave the hospital on.

Necessity does wonders, and since it is necessary for the advertising to be placed and ready to be mailed, Ray J. is back on the job with the aid of his walker. Joan is concerned about the safety of using his left foot for the gas as well as for the brake since his right leg can't be used just yet. He assures her that since his life is at stake, he does drive carefully. Women!

Whenever Joan takes Corinne for her morning ride, she hooks Ray J. up to an alarm in the car in case of an emergency. One day while they are gone, he decides to mow the lawn since it hasn't been mowed for weeks. He can use the lawn mower as a walker, so he takes the alarm off and puts it on the grass. Joan and Corinne hear the alarm go off and just know that he has fallen so they rush back home. Coming in sight of the house, they see the walker where he left it and assume the worst. When they pull into the drive and see him holding onto the handle of the mowing machine, Joan jumps out of the car with,

"I could just break your other hip. You have any idea of how scared you made me?"

Arizona

When the light begins to leave Corinne's eyes, and she complains of being afraid of the dark, of being in a strange town without any of her friends, even afraid of the waiter at her favorite restaurant, they decide they must do what is best for her. After all, she has done what is best for them for as long as they've been married. She is the one who leaves Virg to fend for himself while she comes to California when Heather is born and stays until Joan is able to take care of the baby. She is also the one who leaves Virg again to come to Oklahoma when Derek is due. When the doctor decides he is a month off in the delivery time, she stays another month and looks after them when Derek is born.

They can never repay her for the time, money, and care she gave them during Joan's battles with cancer. And how quickly she loaned them the money to buy the franchise. Many a Christmas would have been bleak without the $1,000, the $2,000 checks that were slipped into a stocking or left on a dresser to find after she leaves.

2000's

Joan packs her clothes and drives out to Arizona where Corinne's older son lives, and where many of her friends have moved to get away from the cold in Colorado.

As everyone knows, women are the shoppers of the world and Joan remains true to her sex. She shops the small town of twenty thousand and finds the perfect house for them. Located on a corner lot, two families can share the living room, dining, kitchen and breakfast room while having separate wings with two bedrooms and bath in each. She calls Ray J. to discuss it, and of course he tells her to buy it; they have always trusted the judgment of each other in real estate deals.

Leaving Corinne with her brother and his wife, Joan returns to help with the mailing that is due in October. She calls the storage company in Loveland to have her mother's furniture delivered to the new house, which means that Joan is running back and forth from Arizona to Texas. They manage to get the December mailing ready to be mailed, and then go "home" to Arizona to spend the Christmas holidays.

Almost exhausted with the buying and getting settled, running back and forth to Texas to help with the business, and expecting her retired brother and his wife to help look after their mother, Joan can't believe the paper her brother hands her. It is labeled: "Itinerary and Black-out Periods for the coming year". They will be in the south of France for the month of January, which is the month for the next mailing. Trying to convince him they would lose their business without some help with Corinne falls on deaf ears.

"Our reservations have been made for months so we couldn't possibly change them now." Furthermore, as his wife points out,

"Aren't you teachers and accustomed to looking after people? Surely you can see that Corinne and her problems will never fit into our lifestyle. Our two kids are finally grown and out of the house. We've looked forward for years to be free to travel."

Living in two houses in two different states with a business to run in one and a woman in the other who requires constant supervision is impossible. Rather a bleak Christmas that year as the family moves their things from Texas. The business dies, and they lose their franchise, leaving them over $100,000 in debt.

On several occasions Ray J. finds Joan weeping as she watches this shell that once housed her mother slowly change from a trim figure to a fat glob of a woman; hair once so well kept by her hairdresser once a week now matted and dirty because she hates to have it combed. What is inside this creature that makes her lie and hide things in the trash can, under the bed, in a drawer, even under the seat of her favorite chair, and then accuse them of stealing them from her? To eat and sleep are her only desires: lots of sweets and hour after hour of sleep.

When incontinence strikes her bladder and bowels, Joan cringes each time Ray J. follows behind her with a bucket and mop. The odor is so strong that it makes Joan vomit to clean it up. Ray J. must have an iron stomach for it doesn't bother him at all.

Humor helps them through the following years as Corinne digresses into throwing her panties into the toilet each time she goes to the bathroom and comes out naked and walks into the kitchen. Joan leads her like a child back into the bathroom and gives her a shower.

Some days are so sad when she remembers some aspects of her life and wonders if she is sick and why is she not in Loveland where she lives. Joan sits beside her and patiently explains how she came to be in Arizona, and now everything is going to be all right. She is safe, and they will see that she is looked after.

Some nights are uneasy when Corinne begins to wander around the house. One night Ray J. and Joan awaken when they hear the garage door opening. Luckily, she has the keys to the wrong car. Joan asks her what she is doing.

"It's such a beautiful day I thought I would go for a drive up through Estes Park."

She thinks she is in Loveland. The next day Ray J. buys door guards and places them high enough so she can't reach them.

One night at 2 AM she snaps on the light in their bedroom and asks,

"Joanie. Where is Virg? Where is your father? He isn't in bed with me, and I've searched the house over and cannot find him."

More and more of Joan's time is spent in explaining over and over how she came to live with them. She prints signs and puts them on each door of the house and on all the appliances so Corinne doesn't have to ask all the time. Each day she takes her for a long drive to keep her busy and to have something to look forward to. Each time she takes her to the Mayo Clinic in Scottsdale for a check-up or have some minor repair made, she takes her for chocolate ice cream as a reward.

To sit and try to get her caught up with what happened yesterday takes so long that suddenly today is here, so they decide to let her live in the "here and now" and forget the past.

Those who can, Teach; Those who can't, Do

Not too many months of this and Ray J. and Joan know they cannot continue for the remainder of her life. Ray J. has always been an early riser from those early years. He applies at Scottsdale Community College to teach English. The department chair is overjoyed to hear that he loves teaching and wants early morning hours. He teaches English 101 at 6, 7, and 8 AM, and gets home in time for Joan to teach Psych. 101 and Developmental Psych. during the midday hours.

What a relief for both of them to be able to get out of the house and teach again and yet not leave Corinne alone at any time.

Colorado

Meanwhile, Anne's husband is playing mind games with her. First, he quits teaching for he says it doesn't pay enough and the long drive to the college wears him out. He tells Heather,

"Anne has such a well-paying job as an officer of the bank that we don't really need the small amount I'm paid."

When he admits to her that he is about $10,000 in debt with plastic and they can clear that up if she would sell the house in town, Anne sells it. She knows he must be embarrassed to have the phone calls that have been coming in for him. Now he can be relaxed and rub her feet when she comes home tired from standing all day. She knows he loves her for he tells her over and over and sometimes smothers her with kisses.

As each member of the family comes to visit, word spreads to the others how bad things are, but no one dares say anything to Anne. She must come to realize this herself. When summer comes and John is out of school, he drives over for a week. These two are still as close as they were growing up so they go to movies, take trips up to Silverton and Purgatory to view the changing colors of the trees, dine in fine restaurants, and take the famous train ride. John senses that something is wrong when her husband spends most of his time on the computer, obviously in chat rooms.

When he leaves her alone to visit his mother in El Paso, Jeff, a young man she had hired for the bank when she first got her job, comes back into town looking for her. They go out to eat and he tells her he has dated other women, but he can't get her out of his mind. Seeing how unhappy she is, he makes her take a good look at how her husband has been using her: thousands of dollars paying his bills for "get rich quick schemes", expensive gadgets for the computer, how many games can one person play. How many gumball machines are still in the garage that were going to make so much money!

When her husband returns home and tries to get into his mind playing games, Anne tells him she no longer loves him and is seeking a divorce. He does all he can to get her to change her mind and stay with him.

The real estate market is at its peak so she has little trouble selling the house and land. Feeling so free with her divorce, she gives him a check for $17,000 because he is broke and without a job.

January 1st brings in a new year and a new life for Anne. She marries Jeff, and they fly to Paris on their honeymoon. Upon their return, they rent a truck, get her furniture out of storage, and move to Denver.

Heather

With her degree in Spanish and her background in the cultures she has been involved in, Heather secures a position in ESL at a community college in El Paso. Joan and Ray J. are afraid to breathe lest she realize she is actually that close to them. They never discourage her from going any place she desires, but it is a relief to know she is safe and close to them. She returns for the second year, and they breathe a little easier.

Derek

Derek graduates from college with a degree in communication, but he is interested in singing. He and Heather have been doing some gigs to help pay their way through school, and he now has a girlfriend, Michelle, majoring in theatre. He and Michelle move to Seattle, Washington, in order to get involved in the theatre.

Little by little and sometimes by leaps and bounds, poor Corinne loses more of reality and recedes into a world of her own. Some days she refuses her medicine and accuses Joan of trying to poison her. Other days she sneaks her pills into a tissue and throws them into the trash. Now she wipes her mouth constantly and each time throws the tissue into the trash. If the trashcan isn't by her side, she drops it to the floor.

One night she sees a neighbor beating his wife and wants to call the police. Next, he calls over and says he is coming over and beat her too. The minute the sun goes down, evil things begin to happen. Joan knows to close the blinds and turn on all the lights, sometimes all night long.

One afternoon she brings a letter to Joan that she had received some time ago and evidently has read anew.

"Joanie, I must have some sort of a problem. I just received this letter from a friend expressing sorry over the death of my sister. Is Helen dead?"

Joan explains that she has a problem with her memory sometimes but not to worry about it.

"Yes, Helen died over a year ago and everyone went to her funeral. Don't you remember? You saw Charlie and Barb with their two kids. Don and his six. All the beautiful flowers. The whole group of us went out to eat."

"Oh, yes. I remember now."

One morning she looks out the window at a mesquite tree in the back yard.

"I remember when we were just young girls, my best friend Zelda and I used to climb that tree. Rocky Ford has such beautiful trees."

If she had her way, she would sleep twenty hours every day. The best way to get her out of bed is to tell her that food is on the table getting cold. Most of the time she comes straight from the bed to the table without washing her hands or combing her hair. Quite a shock the first time, but now almost a habit. Glaring at Ray J. across the table,

"You son of a bitch. Who are you and what are you staring at?"

To break her habit of sleeping so much, one weekend Ray J. and Joan take her to Laughlin for she has always enjoyed the slots. Pushing her into the slot area in her wheelchair is a sight for sore eyes, as she seems to come alive when she hears the noise that indicates she has won.

After Joan checks them into their room, they persuade Corinne to let them take her to the restaurant to eat. Sitting there surrounded by people of various nationalities, colors, and cultures, she raises her head high and announces in a loud voice,

"I'm so glad I'm white and thin!"

She is definitely white since she hasn't been out in the sun for years, but to see someone that fat and out of shape say "I'm thin" is so comical that everyone laughs; it is obvious to them that she is sick. Such is the life of living with someone weaving her way to the other side.

It is a good weekend for everyone although Corinne doesn't remember it. She is living only in the here and now and anything in the past doesn't exist. Joan worries about her. Everything she reads says that her mother still has the ability to feel emotions. Somehow, she should be able to help her with that.

The day finally arrives when Corinne no longer knows anyone in the house. She thinks Ray J. is the handyman so she is forever ordering him around. She thinks Joan is her mother so she wants to argue with her. Heather and Derek call almost daily, partly to check on their grandmother but more and more they are afraid their parents will get so involved looking after her that their own health might be forgotten. They suddenly fly down to see for themselves. Corinne doesn't know who they are, but pretends she does. Derek says,

"Grandma, I bet you have forgotten my name. What is it?"

"You think I would forget my own grandson? Your name is Jeff, of course."

"That's right. You won't ever forget me, will you?

It is obvious she is in the last of the seven stages Jacque addresses in *As You Like It* sans teeth, sans eyes, sans everything.

Recalling how excited she was with the activities in Laughlin, Ray J. and Joan decide the time has come to find a home where she will have more to keep her busy. Joan wants to place her in a new home for the aged just a few blocks from where they live, but Ray J. maintains she should not be close enough for Joan to try to see her every day. It wouldn't be good for either one of them.

Spending days searching for the right one, they find a nationally known home for Alzheimer patients in a town just twenty-one miles away. They assure them they will engage her in daily activities as well as look after her every need. They think $3,500 a month is a little more expensive than the others they have seen, but it will be worth it to know she is well cared for.

For Joan's peace of mind, they set up a weekly schedule. Joan will visit her on Wednesdays, and Ray J. will on Saturdays. Joan finds her doing watercolors a few times, and Ray J. sees her watching television programs with a group. They begin to relax, thinking they have done the right thing. But then one Saturday Ray J. goes over and she is nowhere in sight. He finds an orderly and asks where she might be. She thinks she must be in her room; she hasn't seen her today.

Ray J. steps into her room to be met with the worst odor of urine he has ever smelled. Corinne is in bed with the covers over her head for the smell is too much even for her. Ray J. finds the caregiver for her floor and demands to know why she is in this condition.

"Well, for the past two days she hasn't wanted to get up, so we just let her alone."

He rushes home to tell Joan what he encountered. They search for another home.

The Marriott has homes for the elderly so they check it out. What a beautiful arrangement: Outside appearance exactly like their motels; carpeted hallways, spacious, with pictures on the walls; a library; a reading room; TV room; activity room with modern equipment; dining room just like the motel; and all the rooms in a section on the backside of the motel that have private baths and doors that lead out to an enclosed yard with green grass. Here she can wander in and out of the house and never be lost.

Corinne can live out her days with the thought that she is traveling and staying at the Marriott. For one who loves to travel, *Life can be beautiful* to the end

"Not Sleepless in Seattle"

Getting a few gigs is not enough income for Derek and Michelle; he gets a job at Kinko's and she goes to work in a bookstore. Heather moves to Seattle and gets a position teaching ESL in an International College. Through a friend at work, Derek takes an evaluation test for Adobe Systems Incorporated and scores so high on the problem solving section that they hire him at a very attractive salary.

At International, Heather teaches half time and advises the other half. She takes a different group through the program each semester. Japanese students, mostly female, make up her first group. The next semester, her group is Arab men.

There is no advancement for Heather until she gets a master's degree, so she moves back home to spend the summer and then enroll in the graduate division at the University of Arizona at Tucson.

Many of the courses she has been taking at UW apply to her program so she is getting her degree in August. Always the free spirit, she applies to several countries for a position for fall.

Joan and Ray J. keep hoping something will be available in England or France, but she wants to go to Japan or some place they speak Japanese, or some place where they speak Arabic. She accepts a position in a university in some tiny country in the Persian Gulf.

"Will the Circle Be Unbroken…"

The circle is nearing completion when Lisa weds Sean and moves into an apartment, and Derek and Michelle announce their wedding plans for the coming July 22. Looks like Joan will finally become a grandmother if Derek and Michelle will just hurry things along.

Lisa finally finds the one person who makes her life complete when her son, Griffin, arrives April10th.

Paula II had wondered why one of her breasts had always been smaller than the other. One day she notices they are the same so she and John examine them to find out why. They find a small lump and immediately rush to the doctor to get an expert opinion. He schedules a fine needle aspiration. The dreadful news of cancer chills their spine as they wait again for the removal of her breast.

Chemotherapy treatments have changed drastically since Joan had them years ago. The oncologist assures them she is going to be fine with the success they now have with these treatments. They begin to relax after a few treatments as Paula starts to get her strength back.

One night as she turns in bed, she suddenly screams in pain with her back. Going through the tests takes forever. They finally tell them what they fear most: it has spread to the bone. Taking the latest in pain pills and wearing a pain patch on her arm, Paula takes experimental treatments at the UCLA Medical Center. Encouraged to think they have it in remission, they make plans to attend the wedding in Seattle.

The Wedding Feast

July 22nd is the most exciting and happiest day the family has had in many, many years. Derek and Michelle planned for their wedding for months, and it is everything they dreamed it would be. The eighty invited guests fly in from all parts of the United States, and the pre-wedding activities go exactly as planned.

The week before, the best man and the groomsmen had kidnapped Derek one night (with Michelle in on it) and flew to Oakland to see the Oakland/Seattle baseball game.

As everyone knows, it rains quite frequently in Seattle, and alternate plans were in place just in case. Not a cloud in the sky all day as the guests board the chartered ship, The Emerald Star, and pull out into the waters. With Seattle as the Emerald City, and they are to honeymoon in Ireland, the Emerald Isle, the basic color scheme for the wedding is Emerald green.

Michelle's older brother, Dan, is the officiating minister, Becky, Michelle's sister, is the matron of honor, Heather is the maid of honor, Jeff, Michelle's friend from high school, and Dan's wife, Kim, are the other attendants. Mike, Derek's best friend, as the best man and the three groomsmen dressed in formal black escort the attendants dressed in teal down to the stern of the ship.

Derek and Michelle have written their own vows. With trembling voice he begins to speak his heart, and as he speaks, the tears begin to flow down his face. Michelle wipes the tears on his face as they begin to flow down hers. As the tears keep coming and the words become more emotional, the subtle sobs from the audience begin to be heard. Following his example, Michelle begins to read her heart-felt words, and her brother, the minister, can't stop the tears from flowing down his cheeks.

Ray J. turns and looks behind him at the audience when the sobs become more noticeable. He sees couples looking into each other's eyes and wiping tears from them. They are obviously recalling their own vows or remembering their wedding.

Drying his eyes, he looks at Joan and thinks back, so many years ago, to that day when he told her he didn't want any more children. He looks back at the bride and groom as Derek kisses Michelle and thinks about the times he had looked at him as he was growing up, imagining what he would be when he became a man.

At last, here he is—a thoughtful, sensitive young man who isn't ashamed to show his emotions and cry in public. Spreading his wings at only seventeen, he continues to fly into whatever adventure he seeks. He loves his job, his city, and his wife, not necessarily in that order.

A man who loves his job is a happy man. But Derek knows that making a living is not the same thing as making a life. At such a young age, he already knows that to focus his energies on his family, his work, the needs of others, happiness will find him.

So many toasts are made to the future of this happy couple. Mike expresses it best,

"Derek would ask me from time to time if I thought he and Michelle would ever get married. I always said I thought they would. One day he insists that I tell him why I thought so and I said, 'I have seen you without her'."

Farewell to Paula & Corinne

With all the excitement of cutting the cake, drinking the toasts, and dancing to the variety of tunes, everyone stops and takes notice as Paula and John do the "Turkey Dance". Only Paula and John know it is the last dance for them, and only Paula knows it is the last day she will have some control over pain.

On the way back to California she begins sobbing because she had wanted to see the Butchart Gardens just one more time. Before she can control it, she begins to be wracked with the sobs of knowing she will also never see John again; he will never see her again. John holds her in his arms and quotes once again *The Saddest Words of Tongue and Pen, What Might Have Been, What Might Have Been.*

The oncologist is kind and gentle when she carefully explains where the tumor is located and what is happening to it. At the rate it is spreading, she had only a few weeks to live. She very quickly follows this with the assurance that she will be given medication to ease the pain.

John begins to help Paula in her crossing over to the other side. Each time she mentions the void that will be left here on earth, he reminds her of the joy she will be bringing to the other side where just this summer her friend Alice has been taken after a sudden automobile accident.

"Just think how happy the two of you will be once again dancing and laughing and talking about your lives together since college days at Pepperdine."

When she slips and becomes depressed, he reminds her what a glorious reunion she will have with Paul and Gail who died of cancer.

"Ha Ha Ha. And you thought you could cripple love, shatter hope, corrode faith...."

How fortunate that Paula lived long enough to be a grandmother for a short period of time. Having missed being a mother, she had often told John and the girls how much she looked forward to being a grandmother. Each day as Griffin is placed in the bed beside her, everyone sees the happiness he brings her. Truly, the "circle of life" is evident with the birth and the impending death.

Sudden "black-outs" start, and Paula begs to be allowed to stay at home. John promises her that she can die at home in her own bed, and he will be beside her until the end.

One night John calls his dad and says he cannot give her attention she needs; he cannot leave her alone for a minute. Ray J. still has weeks of summer school to finish for there are no substitutes to take over his classes at this late date. Joan will come out now and he will come later.

Early the next morning, the nurse from the Marriott calls and says Corinne slumped over at the breakfast table, and they have rushed her to the hospital. Ray J. assures Joan there is nothing she can do about it so go on with her packing.

She flies out immediately and soon after the girls come in. Anne arrives later in the day. Paula's sister gets an extended leave from her job and comes in from Texas. Derek and Michelle come down from Seattle and take over the cooking and cleaning. Heather takes leave of absence from the university and flies in from the Emirates.

Earl and Winnie come in from Texas, looking frail and withdrawn. They want to be there for her to the end, but it is so difficult for them. They were in the room with her when she drew her first breath but don't want to be in the room when she draws her last. Surely, there is nothing more difficult in this life than having a child die, no matter what age. To a parent, a child remains a child forever.

Ray J. has to break the news that Corinne dies on the way to the hospital. They all agree that it is best to have her cremated and hold memorial services in Loveland when Joan can be there.

Joan, Heather, and Derek buy the plane tickets and are ready to leave for Loveland when Joan has a sudden feeling, like a "Godly" nudge, that she should stay with Paula. She takes them to the airport and stays behind. She misses her own mother's memorial services, but that is the day that Paula dies.

Paula, dear Paula, has been a class act all her life. As she was in living, so is she in dying. She keeps asking everyone,

"How do I deserve all this love and attention I am getting? I never knew you loved me this much."

They try to keep their worry from her, but it isn't easy. She looks so frail, less than ninety pounds.

"Don't worry. I am not going to cause anyone any trouble. I will just quietly slip away."

One night as she lies quietly upon her bed, the pain suddenly leaves her for a moment, and she feels a peace like none she has ever felt before. She tells John about it and says everything is going to ok.

True to his promise, John is holding one hand and Joan the other when she draws her last breath. *The hardest part of loving is learning to let go*

Heather and Derek later give them the details of their grandmother's memorial service: They attend the memorial services and then try to find Corinne's ashes. They are told that as a service, her ashes have been "dropped off". They take them out to the cemetery. When the workmen finish digging the grave, they pour her ashes into it. Derek makes the following remarks:

> I am here to say a few words on behalf of my mother about Grandma. There isn't any good way for me to capture what to say on Mom's behalf, because I don't think there are words that could do an adequate job. So, instead, I will share a couple of lessons that Grandma taught me. While I learned a lot from or through Grandma, two things stand out in particular. First, it is important in this life to take care of each

other; and second, respect for those around you should be a part of your daily thoughts.

Mom couldn't be here because she is helping in the care of my sister-in-law who is terminally ill. And we all know that in Grandma's later years she needed a lot of care. Several people gave up a lot and spent a great deal of time and energy with and for Grandma. I know that Mom put in a huge amount of effort to the care of her mother. And she did so, not because she felt obligated, as a child should to a parent, but because Grandma inspired that within her.

Grandma was kind and sweet and generous,

But most importantly, she had a quality that made those that knew and loved her want to be kind and sweet and generous. That is a powerful legacy.

Grandma was the type of person who not only said and thought kind things, but she also did kind things. She acted upon her kindness. And in a life when we are judged by our actions more than our words, this a huge lesson to learn.

Grandma's kindness to me (among other things) was to help teach me respect. I have bad hair. I have tried to fight this fact for years, but there is no denying, my hair is goofy. So because of this, you will be hard pressed to see me without a hat on my head. It is a kind of fixture. When I was going to school in Greeley, and Grandma was living in Loveland, I would come over on occasions to dinner. I'd pick up Grandma and we would go to the Red Lobster, sit down, and she would tell me to remove my hat. I would object and she would tell me that I should remove my hat because to do so is polite and respectful, especially in the presence of ladies.

This was the pattern. I would pick up Grandma, we would sit down, and she would tell me to remove my hat because to do so was polite and respectful especially in the presence of ladies.

One weekend, Heather and the girl who would become my wife and I went to Grandma's house for dinner. We sat down, and I quickly removed my hat. Now at this time I thought I would be cool if I grew out my hair. Somehow, if it was long, I thought it would be less goofy. Grandma looked at me and said, "Boy, what is the matter with your head?" When I protested, she told me that I looked like a Troll-doll...only Troll dolls were cuter. I was flabbergasted and everyone was laughing. Then it hit me that you can be polite and respectful, but you can also be relaxed and have a good time.

So that is what I learned from Grandma. I try to take care of the people I love and who love me, and I try to show them respect without being uptight. So, today, I wear no hat, Grandma. And when I sit down to a nice dinner, I remove my hat because to do is polite and respectful, especially in the presence of ladies.

I love you, Grandma, and I miss you. And I know the only reason that Mom is not here today is because she is following your example. *The hardest part of loving is learning to let go.*

So many friends of Paula's from school come by with their words of praise for Paula and how much she will be missed. Neighbors with pies and cakes and goodies pour in so fast they have to be scheduled in order to get into the house.

At the service for Paula, Joan reads the following:

"Ray J. Pharr, John's father and patriarch of the family, couldn't be here today, but he wanted this to be shared. It is an email that he sent to the family upon hearing about Paula's critical condition. 'The Wonderful Trip' he refers to occurred when he was returning home after being treated for prostate cancer and was contemplating his own death.
Hi all,
Something I've been thinking about ever since that wonderful trip Joan and I made to Denver, especially the trip back home. As a society, we have robbed ourselves, we have frightened our children, and we have made ourselves miserable with the word 'death'. I know the Bible says we should cry at a birth and rejoice at a death, but we have reversed it. The real truth is that we are miserable because we are going to miss that person. The closer we get to that age or circumstance when we finally give in and say, "Yes, it will happen to me", we then begin to see the big picture a little more closely. I find it hard to think of being in the presence of my Maker and all the loved one and friends who have gone on before me and being a part of their lives and at the same time thinking of how I will miss those who are still on earth. But, it won't be that long, in terms of eternity, until they, too, will be joining us, and that is the makeup of the Kingdom of God. After all, we are spirit, and when we are joined with so many spirits of God, it is no wonder there is great rejoicing in Heaven when one more spirit comes home. Just think, at a time when we are sad, weeping, and thinking how much we are going

to miss Paula, she is the happiest she has ever been—safe, secure, no more pain, no more sadness, finally getting the answers to all the questions she has ever had".

Hope Springs Eternal

The first year passes and the circle continues. John immediately goes back to work and the routine of life. He spends most of the first months in going to work each morning, coming home in time to eat, and then writing "Paula's Story". He and Paula had talked about his ability to write during her last weeks. She wanted him to let others know about her plight and hoped the telling of it would help those who might pass this way.

He sells the house at the beach which is too full of memories and buys a beautiful home near his teaching grounds. Now, he gets to work in fifteen minutes with no freeways, no frantic drivers trying to get to work one car ahead of the other, and returns home the same way.

Anne and Jeff, who have moved to Beaumont, Texas, in order for Jeff to go back to school to become an audiologist, run out of funds when their house in Denver won't sell. Anne tries for months to find a position but there a re none available.

When John hears of their plight, he offers a suggestion:

"Here I am all alone in this big house and don't use half of it. There is a whole wing with two bedrooms and bath plus the sitting room on the other side of the hall. Why don't you two move out here? Jeff can go to school at one of the universities in downtown LA which is less than half an hour from here".

They jump at the chance. Loading their furniture in a large truck and moving for days through the desert is exhausting. In a matter of days, they place their furniture in storage and settle into being at home with John. Anne searches the want ads for work and finds nothing. She pays her dues to an agency to find her a position. She waits for something to turn up. Jeff is taking courses that run for a few weeks and then full time for summer.

Lisa, Sean, and Griffin move into the other bedroom so Lisa can continue her education to become an elementary teacher. Already the house abounds with the busy members reading, writing, studying, and getting on with life. The one common denominator that keeps them all together, focused on the future and its promise, is Griffin. He is now walking and running and smiling bringing such joy to so many people.

Rachael, John's younger daughter, and Jordie, her partner in physical therapy work as well as in life, get married and buy a home in San Luis Obispo, only hours from John and the family.

John is taking dancing lessons and slowly moving back into the social world. Friends from work take him to eat, to Los Vegas, to small parties. Each day brings him closer to finishing "The Paula Story", and each day the pain of losing her grows dimmer.

Heather is on her way home for the summer. She has one more year to fulfill her contract, and then she is off to parts unknown. Something has been said about Spain, but no one knows exactly that that means, not even Heather. The family smiles and waits. Heather is well known for her sudden change of plans. How many plane tickets have been changed at the last moment? How much money has she spent in making changes no one dare keep tab.

Another unknown with Heather is the "Brit" she has been seeing and the one who is coming home with her. What is known is that she will never move permanently to another country and leave her beloved family as well as her country.

Ray J. and Joan can hardly wait for their "wanderer" to get home once more. She is the "gypsy" part of them that is eager to move and want more and more out of life. She is just beginning a life that will be full of experiences neither of them have had.

EPILOGUE

Well, son. I know I have rambled somewhat in my thinking, but I think I have covered what I wanted to share. You best just tell your daughter about our past. This is just between us men and not for ladies to read.

It has been good for Joan and me to write down pretty much our life story. We have been remembering the wonderful life we have shared. *Winters must be cold for those who have no warm memories.*

One of the things that stands out at the moment is that one should always leave loved ones with loving words because one day it will be the last time they will be seen.

Also, with fourscore behind me, I realize it has taken me a long time to become the person I want to be. But, *I have miles to go before I sleep. Miles to go before I sleep.*

Some days I am the pigeon; some days I am the statue.

0-595-34358-9

www.ingramcontent.com/pod-product-compliance
Lightning Source LLC
Chambersburg PA
CBHW020239290526
45784CB00003B/1041